W9-AYN-845

praise for
Food Guilt No More

"When we grow up experiencing the opposite of love—indifference, rejection, and abuse—we become addicts in search of feelings we never experienced in a healthy way. Information does not fix the problem, but inspiration and self-esteem do.

"Lindsey's book faces both these issues and provides us with a guidebook to a healthier and happier life. When you change your life experience, everything else falls into place.

"In heaven, the vegetarian, meditating joggers are very bitter about all the time they spent trying not to die and never having time to love their chocolate ice cream. So read on and learn to make your life a delicious meal while giving your body the gift of a healthier life."

—Bernie Siegel, MD, author of *Peace, Love, and Healing*

"This book is a game-changer for emotional eaters. Lindsey shines a compassionate light on food guilt and makes the journey fun for the reader. I would recommend this book to anyone looking to overhaul their relationship with food."

—Heather Waxman, author of *BODYpeace*

"Many people today suffer from the pain of food guilt. Lindsey Smith has been working with clients one on one, and now she's written a book addressing this topic so her advice and inspiration will be available to people around the world. If you have been trying different diets or feeling guilt and shame about food, this book is for you."

—Joshua Rosenthal, founder of the Institute for Integrative Nutrition

Food Guilt No More

TAME YOUR CRAVINGS AND EAT YOUR WAY TO HAPPINESS

Lindsey Smith

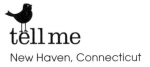

tell me

New Haven, Connecticut

This book is for general instruction only; it is not a medical manual. The information in this book is not intended to replace or interrupt the relationship with or treatment from a physician or other professional. If you are pregnant or breast-feeding, are under a doctor's care for any reason, or suspect you have a medical problem, consult your doctor before beginning this or any program. The author, editors, and publisher are not responsible for errors or omissions or for any application of the information in this book and make no warranty, either implied or expressed, with regard to this edition or future editions of the content of this book.

Mention of specific products, companies, organizations, or authorities in this book does not imply endorsement by the author or publisher, nor does their mention imply that they endorse this book, its author, or its publisher.

Copyright © 2015 by Lindsey Smith

All rights reserved. No part of this book may be reproduced or transmitted in any form or by any electronic or mechanical means, including information storage and retrieval systems, without permission in writing from the publisher.

To my dad, who taught me
the power of cooking

Contents

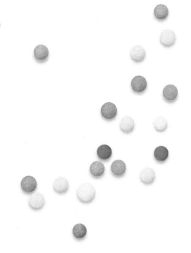

Acknowledgments

Much gratitude to the many friends and supporters who have been by my side since the birth of *Junk Foods and Junk Moods*. Without you, this book would not be possible.

I would also like to thank my amazing editor, Paula Brisco, who made this book shine and totally got my style from day one.

To my publishing team: thank you for believing in me and working with me so closely and authentically on this project.

Introduction

In the United States, 79 percent of women—and 65 percent of men—experience food guilt, according to a 2015 Harris Poll. That's a lot us of grappling with feelings of uneasiness, shame, anxiety, fear, stress, and unhappiness over what we put on our fork.

Food guilt can cause us to overeat, undereat, or develop dysfunctional relationships with food. It can take the pleasure out of mealtimes or gatherings with friends. It can lead us to hide snack stashes or sneak-eat in the car or tiptoe downstairs in the wee nighttime hours for a guilty serving of our latest indulgence.

I'm here to tell you that life doesn't have to be this way. It's time to relinquish food guilt and learn to love your meals and yourself.

I speak from firsthand experience. Food guilt paralyzed me for years. Whether I ate kale or cookies, broccoli or brownies, I agonized over meals as well as treats. Eventually, I recognized food guilt's sneaky symptoms and built my program to tame cravings, find foods that energize and sustain, and break the guilt cycle. *In Food Guilt No More*, I share the program with you.

My journey away from food guilt began, oddly enough, with a picnic.

Picnic Guilt

"Are you coming to the picnic with me next week, Lindsey?" Zach asks enthusiastically.

Hesitantly, I answer, "Eh, I don't know yet. I want to, but we'll see."

"Well, you should come—it'll be so much fun," Zach replies. "I'm really excited! There will be lots of food and good people."

I try to respond with excitement, but I can't muster more than a fake smile and a wimpy, "Yeah, it will be great" line.

Immediately after I receive Zach's invitation, my palms sweat and my stomach turns in knots. I think to myself, *Fun? Yeah, I'm sure fun is the exact word for you. For me, a picnic is more like torture.*

I should be eager to join a festive outing with friends, but I'm suddenly stressed and depressed. In place of excitement, I have dread. It's not that I don't want to see friends or hang around a campfire—I do enjoy those things.

The stress I feel is one I bury deep inside me: food stress.

To me, a picnic means much more than playing horseshoes and joining in campfire conversations. Despite my best efforts to keep things in balance, picnics are all about struggles with food.

So the minute Zach mentions "picnic," I immediately think, *Oh no—fattening pasta salad, thigh-enhancing cookies, and love-handle brownies.*

What excuse can I give to not attend the picnic? My mind goes blank; no excuse is good enough. I realize I must suck it up and attend this "fun" event.

For an entire week, I remain food stressed: *Should I starve myself before or after the cookie bingeing? Can I exercise for two hours before the picnic to preburn the calories? Maybe I should get up extra early the next morning and do hot yoga to sweat out all the fat and sugar I will have inhaled.* I think of everything and anything to keep off the weight I am sure to gain.

Then the mental guilt kicks in. *Why me?* I scream inside my mind. I think I am probably the only person stressing about food before a party even begins. I want to be normal. I want to enjoy food. I want to feel good. I just want to get rid of all this FOOD GUILT!

After a week of torment and stress, I arrive at the picnic. I smell meat cooking on the grill. My stomach grumbles. I starved myself all day in preparation for this event and told myself I won't indulge. This time, for once, I will have the willpower I need to resist!

But my stomach is aching, and I am seriously on the verge of tears. I want to eat; I don't want to eat. The internal dialog is killing me. I am pretending to be present, pretending to care what my friends are saying, pretending to have fun, while the entire time I am engaged in this invisible mental fencing match. Just as I think I am winning the match, my opponent ducks and comes at me from a different angle. I see food. I smell food. I am overwhelmed by the urge to eat.

I make my way past the plethora of breads and pasta salads. *Hurrah*, I think, *the temptations are coming to an end.* For a moment I have a sense of relief. The food is not going to win this time!

Then I halt. The dessert table is directly in front of me. Cookies, brownies, cakes, pies, bonbons, whoopie pies—you name the sugary substance, it is on this table. My mouth waters. My stomach pains become more pronounced.

The mental sparring resumes.

"You know you shouldn't have that brownie, Lindsey. Just think what it will do to your thighs!"

"But I just want *one*. One won't hurt me, right?!"

"DON'T DO IT!!! Stay away from the chocolate cake! Have more willpower than that! Don't fail now!"

"But I just want one . . ."

This battle has worn me out. I managed to skip the pasta and bypass the bread, but the brownies, the cakes, the cookies—no, I can't resist anymore.

I give in. I scarf down a brownie in seconds. After a few moments of pleasure, I sit back, realizing that I have just been defeated.

I can't believe I did that! Any sense of willpower is gone. I feel so ashamed, so guilty. A failure. In my battle with food, food has just won.

So I embrace my shame and misery and proceed to fill a plate with sugary goodies. Since I've already done the damage, I might as well drown in my own sweet misery. Literally!

At home that evening, I crash from the sugar rush, feeling depressed and lethargic. I sleep fitfully, thinking about how I couldn't enjoy myself like everyone else at the picnic. I was there physically, but my mind was elsewhere. I barely remember the conversations or the people. I was so fixated on food, I couldn't allow the friendships and fun times to nourish me in a way that a chocolate brownie never could. Lying awake, I wonder why I continuously live in this fear of food. I feel a prisoner to my pantry.

Saying Good-Bye to Picnic Guilt . . . and Other Kinds of Food Guilt

For years, I reenacted versions of that picnic scenario. For years, food guilt was my constant companion, robbing me of enjoyment, tarnishing my relationships, depleting my self-image, and threatening my physical and mental health. One day, however, I thought, *There has to be another way.* Although I kept my food guilt hidden, I knew I wasn't the only person who struggled. If I were the only one, there wouldn't be a new diet craze each year! But I didn't want a diet. I wanted to know why I and others struggle with guilt *and fear* surrounding food. I wanted a sustainable and satisfying relationship with food.

I determined to find that better path—and I did. Although I can't say my relationship with food is always smooth sailing now, I can say that the battle no longer dominates my life. Today, my approach to food is most often characterized by love rather than guilt. I'm happy and healthy. I eat with appreciation and enjoyment. And I've found a rewarding career as the Food Mood Girl—holistic health coach, motivational speaker, and author. I work with people like you (and me!) to transform their relationship with food.

While writing my first book, *Junk Foods and Junk Moods*, I coined the "recipe to health and happiness." This formula served as the foundation for my work. It's how I helped my clients and readers overcome the "junk food and junk mood" cycle. The principles are simple:

Think good thoughts. Eat real food. Love yourself. Repeat as necessary.

Once I started meeting more people through my book tour and speaking engagements, however, I realized that people were still struggling with emotional eating, stress eating, and food/mood imbalances. Women (and men!) came up to me at events and said, "I know cupcakes are bad for me, but sometimes I just want one, you know?" Others would say, "I love chips a lot. Is it that bad?"

There was one connection to all their concerns—food guilt.

So I decided to get to the root cause of what was causing such guilt and why people were unable to break the negative cycle. Through my research and encounters, I noticed something shocking. *This guilt wasn't just happening with emotional eaters, it was happening with colleagues as well.* Health coach friends and professionals would experience guilt for days about eating a nonorganic apple or feel reprehensible because they went out for ice cream during a family vacation. Even bananas were making people cringe because of the media hype about their "high sugar content."

From this has come my new formula, the Food Freedom Paradigm. It's similar to my recipe for health and happiness, except it adds one crucial component: *eat with love.* I believe that if people feel good about what they are eating, they will have less guilt and shame and therefore experience fewer binges and negative emotions attached to food. Here's the new Food Freedom Paradigm in graphic form.

Food Freedom Paradigm

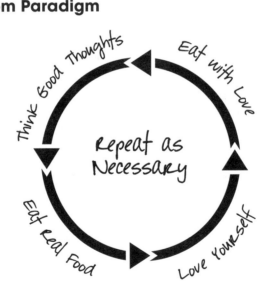

The paradigm works. Over time, I have seen the shift in clients and heard testimonials during speaking engagements and on my blog. Shifting your perspective on food, it turns out, is essential for good health—and happiness.

How to Use This Book

With this new emphasis on eating with love, I created this book to encompass more than just lists of what to eat and not to eat. I wrote a fun, inspirational, and often personal guide that shares recipes and takes the guilt and fear out of food and transforms it into love—all in the kitchen.

My motto is:

If you want a cupcake, eat it and feel really damn good about it.

So, yes, while *Food Guilt No More* features recipes, it is so much more than a cookbook. Use it to learn how to overcome intense cravings and find the best food solutions to improve your mood. Explore the sections on how to treat your body like a test lab—in the positive sense of finding just the right foods to sustain *your* individual needs. Above all, learn the techniques that support my Food Freedom Paradigm. Best of all, the soul-satisfying recipes adhere to this paradigm. They go beyond physical nourishment and truly transform how you view yourself and your body. And, of course, these delicious recipes and tips will help you truly love and appreciate your food.

True health transformation—overcoming food guilt, taming your cravings, and eating your way to happiness—starts in the kitchen, the heart of the home.

In these pages, I share what I've learned from my own journey, and from those of my clients, so that you, too, can replace food guilt with food love—regardless of if the food is kale or a cupcake!

Let's get cookin' and lovin'!

1

Why We Feel Deprived

ood guilt. How can so many of us be surrounded by food yet still feel deprived? Why are we afraid of a dessert? Why do we go through "eating agony"? Why do we feel such shame that we can't even admit our obsession with food?

I define food guilt as the guilt we feel around eating or not eating certain foods. Especially when it comes to eating "junk food" or falling off the healthy-eating wagon.

Whether it's spurred by a picnic, a co-worker's birthday celebration, or that treat drawer where we keep things hidden, the food guilt we experience is real. And often it seems like a song that repeats over and over.

Those of us who experience food guilt tend to see food in terms of black and white; good and bad; calories in and calories out. We immediately feel defeated when we eat something we've labeled as "bad" or when we consume calories beyond the government or media hype recommendations. We fret about our food choices at home, at work, and at social gatherings. We think about what new diet we can start tomorrow to compensate for today's cake and ice cream. Negative food thoughts crowd our minds, making it hard to focus on much else.

When it comes down to it, of course, we need food to live. So how do we meet our needs and get around food guilt so we can live healthy, happy lives? How can we experience food in a way that frees us from the guilt hangover? How can we choose meals and recipes that nourish us physically and emotionally? It starts by recognizing that food is meant to be enjoyed.

Nutrition, Needs, Cravings, and Emotional Eating

People crave and eat in response to nutritional needs. Not all needs, however, can be met through food. As people with bodies, minds, and spirits, we require various types of nourishment, including good food, positive relationships, and spiritual sustenance.

We get in trouble and begin a cycle of food guilt when we try to satisfy cravings of the mind and spirit with food. The problem isn't simply that we choose "bad" foods, it's that we choose food as our nutrient of choice, no matter what the need.

Foods, especially foods with high sugar or fructose content, offer temporary satisfaction and even a brief high that allow us to escape the pain and longings we feel. Unfortunately, if the underlying emotional issues or needs are left unresolved, our temporary satisfaction is quickly followed by food guilt and self-disgust.

I coach clients who think of themselves as emotional eaters, those who are plagued with food guilt. I help them identify their deeper underlying issues when it comes to food. For example, some people:

- Suffer from the fear of "not having enough" because food was scarce growing up.

- Use food as a coping mechanism or a type of self-protection because they don't want to be taken advantage of.

- Eat due to stress.

- Eat to fill a deeper void of self-hate, thinking that somehow the chocolate bar might love them back.

- Have a deep fear of not connecting with others—a feeling of being alone, unsupported, unappreciated, and/or unloved.

Whatever the cause may be, we eat for all kinds of reasons.

And let's face it: anyone who struggles with food, myself included, has a story of fear, heartache, neglect, or abuse.

My own cycle of emotional eating began when I was in preschool. At the end of each preschool day, the teachers would take us students outside to wait for our parents. Each parent would drive up displaying a bright yellow or neon green laminated sign with a child's name. The teacher or teacher's assistant would then take the child to the parent's car, and the family would drive away.

Day after day, I'd watch each of my peers escorted to a car displaying a sign. Joey, Jocelyn, Lauren, Paul, and the others were all picked up. A young child's eternity would go by, and still there was no sign for me. Feelings of anxiety would arise. *Where are my parents? Are they okay? Did they forget about me?*

My parents, struggling to manage the responsibilities of a retail store, were frequently late. But as a child, I didn't comprehend those obligations. As I waited, I'd fidget, worry, and grow anxious and despondent. By the time my mom or dad showed up, I'd feel forgotten, neglected, hurt, and lost. It happened over and over.

One particular day, my mom showed up last—again. The moment I saw her, I started sobbing. Tears poured out. I began to scream. I couldn't calm down. In a desperate attempt to stop my hysteria, my mom did the only thing she thought would work. She took me to Don Mann's, a local convenience store filled with penny candy.

Mom told me to pick out any candy I wanted. The bright colors and the rows of jars were enough to distract and excite me, and my tears dried. I filled my little brown paper bag with all the essentials: watermelon gummies, Sour Patch gummies, red Swedish fish, flying saucers.

This interplay of emotions and consoling food became a routine. Every time my parents were late, I was rushed off to get a quick sugar fix to make it all better. My parents were treating my junk mood with junk food.

This routine set me up at a young age for an unhealthy relationship with food. I began to associate feelings of hurt, neglect, and sadness with cravings for sweets to comfort me. It seemed these foods could take away any negative feelings I had, at least temporarily. The candy, of course, was never able to address the real problem—my need to be loved and remembered. Not knowing or understanding the connection, I became an emotional eater and a food guilt sufferer.

When all the extra eating showed in my weight during my teen years, I felt different and unattractive. When I began to try to lose the weight, however, I discovered that food—my temptress—was everywhere.

As anyone who tries to stick to a diet or lose weight knows, food is frequently at the center of human connection. Food is social and emotional. When we want to celebrate, we gather and serve food. When we need to grieve, we gather and serve food. As human beings, we crave connections, especially through friendships and other relationships. Food often brings us together—for gatherings, celebrations, holidays, and events.

So we eat the brownie to join in the gathering but also because we believe it will bring a feeling of indulgence and satisfaction, no matter how short-lived. But for those of us with food guilt, the guilt and shame we feel for eating a brownie makes us uncomfortable and exacerbates the ways in which we see ourselves as different, the ways in which we believe we don't fit or belong. Our failure with food seems to symbolize everything wrong with us.

If this cycle continues, we no longer enjoy the celebration, picnic, or outing with friends. We feel distant from the people we love. We feel bad for caring more about food than about each other. We fear that if people knew our deep dark secrets, they wouldn't like us anymore. We fear that if people see us eat that extra slice or two of pizza or that fourth brownie, they might not want to associate with us.

At the end of the day, we all want to relate, be connected, and belong. We want to feel loved and appreciated. We want to enjoy our communal events and enjoy the food that comes along with it. We want to be nourished in relationships as well as in mind, body, and spirit.

What about you? What are your underlying food guilt triggers? Here's an exercise to help you dig a little further into your cravings and true hungers.

Make a list of the things you crave. List the foods you crave, but also list the deeper things. Which cravings belong to relationships? the mind? the body? the spirit? Don't be afraid to go deep.

_____

_____

_____

_____

_____

_____

Next, list some nonfood ways you can nourish your relationships, your body, your mind, and your spirit.

_____

_____

_____

_____

_____

_____

Meet My Lindsey-isms!

Oftentimes when speaking or writing, I use words or phrases that initially need a little explanation. Here are the Lindsey-isms you'll meet in this book.

Cook with love (v): To cook with good energy; to put love into everything you make.

Eat with love (v): To love your food, whether it's a piece of kale or a cookie; to practice eating with good energy.

Food guilt (n): The guilt we feel around eating or not eating certain foods—especially when it comes to eating "junk food" or falling off the healthy-eating wagon.

Food hangover (n): When you binge on so much food that the entire night and next morning you feel like you got run over by a truck.

Hangry (adj): When you are so hungry, you become angry.

Junk mood (n): A type of mental state after eating junk food or thinking negative thoughts.

Real food (n): You know, the stuff that comes from the ground or grows on trees, not processed in a lab. Oh yeah, you should also be able to pronounce it.

Repalling (adj): It's so repulsive, it's appalling.

Rewrite Your Food Story
to Decrease the Power of Food Guilt

You can start breaking free from food guilt by rewriting your personal food story. The idea is to stop using food as a scapegoat for not connecting in the way you wish. Instead, identify the connection you crave and rewrite your story to fit just that. For example:

Current Story

Food is the thing I constantly think about. I am always obsessing about my next meal or sugary snack. I want my relationship with food to be normal and to be able to stop when I am no longer hungry or to stop at one piece of candy or one cookie.

I know people judge me for how I eat and how overweight I am. If I can just get control over what I eat, every part of my life will be better.

New Story

Food provides essential nutrients for my body. My relationship with food IS enjoyable and satisfying. I am learning to eat when I am hungry and to stop when I am full. I am filling my mind with good thoughts when it comes to food. I am learning to enjoy the tastes and nourishment that food provides.

I am more than my body, and I need nutrients beyond food. I choose to nourish myself by reaching out to friends and family members. I am spending time with positive and encouraging people rather than those who criticize me. I choose to nourish my spiritual self with walks, meditation, and church. As I make progress in nourishing the physical, relational, and spiritual aspects of myself, my life is improving.

Here's another example:

Current Story

I hate the fact that I have no control over food. Candy is my weakness. I eat for every emotion—happy, sad, anxiety, and guilt. It all started when I was twelve and felt neglected and hurt. I want to get my food intake under control, but it's so hard. The bad things that happened when I was twelve set a pattern in motion. I'm not strong enough to fix it. Let's face it: I'm a failure. Maybe I can try that new diet I just heard about. . . .

New Story

I developed some bad habits around food, but it is possible to change. I'm ready to talk about and face the painful things that happened when I was twelve, perhaps with a coach or professional counselor. I need to heal so that my coping mechanism, food, has a less powerful pull for me.

Although I am hurting, I know I have strengths and that I am enough. I don't have to have an all-or-nothing relationship with food. I can choose foods that nourish me without going to a negative extreme. I don't have to live a life of deprivation. Rather than wallow in my mistakes and failures, I am adding sources of enrichment and nourishment to my life. For example, I now spend time with friends for a walk in the park or a drive to the country.

Notice how the new stories are written in a positive, achievement-based voice—"I will," "I am," "I do." They speak in the present tense so that the new story is framed in actions today, not steps postponed until tomorrow. Review the two examples again. Now rewrite your own story.

Your Current Story

_____

_____

_____

_____

_____

Your New Story

_____

_____

_____

_____

_____

Now breathe. Take in your new story and feel good about it. Read it every single day as you start your journey to rid yourself of constant food guilt and nourish yourself with love and patience. Refer to it as you select foods, as you choose recipes and make your meals. Make your new story come alive!

I realize this is easier said than done. Yet, sharpening your resolve can help you banish food guilt for good. Anytime you experience food guilt, remember that you have the opportunity to revise or rewrite your food story as needed.

With your new story and sense of direction in hand, let's learn to cook with love!

2

Bring Positive Energy and Love to Your Food

Did you know that you don't simply take nutrients and energy *from* food, you also bring a certain amount of energy *to* your experience with food?

When we allow ourselves to sink into constant guilt about eating something we think we shouldn't, we create negative energy. When we feel anxious about eating a cookie, we end up obsessing and stressing over the cookie before, during, and after we actually eat it. This ultimately puts unnecessary stress on our bodies and minds as we eat and digest that little treat.

Can you think of a time when you experienced butterflies in your stomach, perhaps when you were anxious or stressed about giving a speech or completing a project? That's because 95 percent of your body's stress hormones sit in your gut, making your stomach the first responder to stress, hence the fluttering butterflies.

Any type of stress (good or bad) causes your body to move into a state of fight or flight. During this state, your body regears to focus on three things: fight off an attacker, run to get away, and think clearly to calculate its next move. The last thing your body focuses on in this moment is digesting food. So when you are stressing about the cookie, the flight-or-fight response triggers—then bam! You probably experience indigestion, acid reflux, and an upset stomach along with your guilty conscience.

Your body cannot distinguish between the stress you feel in a medical emergency and the stress you feel from eating a bag of cookies. In either case, the stress makes it harder on your body to digest what you eat. This is how stress (including food guilt and weight guilt) often leads to constipation, bloating, acid reflux, and even weight gain.

You can influence the amount of stress your body has to deal with by altering your attitude toward food. Stop thinking of food in terms of "good" or "bad" and start bringing positive energy toward food choices. If you are going to eat a cookie, appreciate and enjoy the cookie.

I designed four simple steps, described below, to put more positive energy into your food and, in turn, your life. Try cooking with love, eating with love, creating a personal mantra, and meditating on an eating experience.

Step 1: Cook with Love

Whenever you cook a meal, pour extra helpings of love into it. And no, I am not talking about a magic "love" spice you can sprinkle on. I'm talking about sprinkling on loving, positive, calming, centered, or cheerful energy while cooking.

Some folks think this sounds wacky or a bit too earthy-crunchy. (I admit, I have to watch my hippie tendencies.) But it's not! Remember that the theory of positive intention has a long and storied history. Norman Vincent Peale wrote a best seller in 1952 called *The Power of Positive Thinking*. Oprah Winfrey has built her career around choosing an attitude of gratitude. Attitude counts, in food and in life.

Figure out what energy you want to experience and cook with that energy. Do you want your meal to be a calming, energizing, or a peaceful experience? Visualize the end result and give each pour, scoop, stir, mix, and sauté the exact energy you want to get out of your experience.

You have the ability to add feelings of love, gratitude, and bliss into your food by transferring your energy to it. Dance while you are sautéing, sing while you are mixing, or simply listen to the radio and smile!

It doesn't matter whether you are preparing boxed mac 'n' cheese or crafting a homemade version; regardless of the food's nutritional value, cook with a positive and blissful energy. Not only will you have more fun in the kitchen, you'll also appreciate what you are eating, digest your food better, and even eat less because you get "full" on your energy.

Cook with your best attitude, and good energy will return to you.

 Food Mood Girl Mantra: Create an affirmation to use while cooking. Each recipe in this book suggests an affirmation. But if you have an affirmation that sounds special to you, then cook with that one. Examples: *I am blissful. I am loving. I am kind. I accept myself.*

Step 2: Eat with Love

Whether you make one of the recipes in this book or purchase a meal, bring positive energy to your eating. Many times, we feel so shameful about what we are consuming that we can barely focus on anything else. We end up berating ourselves for wanting or eating something we think of as "bad." Other times, we eat mindlessly, in haste, barely acknowledging hunger or satiation. When we put negative energy and emotion into our food, this energy shows up in our bodies as negative moods, low energy, and low self-esteem.

Instead of going into your eating experience with traumatic, stress-inducing thoughts, eat with a state of love and appreciation. I don't care if you choose fast food, convenience food, or farm-fresh food. Enter each relationship with food in a state of love, gratitude, and appreciation.

Your food will not only digest better, but you will feel better about eating it.

Step 3: Create a Personal Mantra

Creating a personal mantra is a great way to keep yourself in check or to lovingly remind yourself to calm down when you are feeling a bit crazed. Next time you are at a gathering and you get caught up with food anxiety, say one of these short mantras—or craft a mantra of your own to help you overcome the food guilt moment. A mantra can put your body in a calm state so you feel less tense about food choices.

My Personal Mantras

1. When it comes to food, I choose love.
2. Whether I choose kale or a cookie, I will eat it with love.
3. I will eat this _____ , and my body will use it for good.
4. I nourish my mind, body, and spirit with nutrients that match my real cravings.
5. This food will nourish me in positive ways.
6. I am enough.
7. I nourish my mind and spirit as well as my body.

Your Personal Mantras

1. _____

2. _____

3. _____

4. _____

5. _____

6. _____

7. _____

Step 4: Meditate on the Food Experience

When we label sweet, sour, or salty flavors as "bad" food, we set ourselves up for misery. That's because when we eat self-declared bad foods, we feel like failures. Then we console ourselves by eating more of the very foods we've been trying to avoid.

You can break out of this cycle by meditating while you eat something you crave. Meditating on your food is a great way to savor its flavors, colors, smells, textures, and sounds. You'll expand your palate so you can taste food more fully and increase your sense of satisfaction. You'll gain a healthy pleasure in what you eat and resist the impulse to consume multiple helpings. In short, you will enjoy your food more.

Here's a sample exercise.

Mini Chocolate Meditation

Begin with a bar of dark chocolate (or other food of choice). Feel the packaging. Listen to the crinkle or other sounds the wrapper makes as you open it. Look closely at the ridges and markings on the chocolate bar.

Break off a piece of the chocolate. Breathe in the strong cocoa aroma. Notice how your body reacts. Is your mouth watering? Are you feeling calm, relaxed, or tense?

Lick the piece of chocolate. Again, pay attention to sensations in your body. Now take a small bite and keep the chocolate on your tongue. How does it feel? Is it melting quickly or slowly? Pay attention to textural changes. Keep focused on how your body reacts.

As the chocolate melts, swallow it and follow its movement into your stomach. Continue noticing the sensations in your body. Repeat the meditation process until the chocolate is gone.

What do you notice from this exercise? Was the chocolate more satisfying? Did you find more pleasure in the treat? Could you stop at just one piece?

Treat Your Body as a Test Lab

Just as you bring positive or negative energy to your food, the foods you eat bring positive or negative energy to you. When you eat an apple, your body reacts in one way. When you eat an ice-cream cone, your body reacts differently. What's more, your body is unique in its reactions. How your body responds to an apple will be different from how my body reacts to that same variety of apple.

When it comes to smart food choices, experiment and listen to your own body. Don't worry about what foods work for me or for someone else. Treat your body as a test lab. When you drink coffee, what is your body's reaction? When you eat broccoli, how does your body feel? When you eat something made of white flour, how does your body respond? When you consume a huge brownie sundae, what is the result? After each food, observe your energy level. Notice how your stomach feels—comfortable or bloated. Pay attention to headaches, mood swings, or other reactions. Keep a journal of your findings.

As you listen to your body's responses to foods, pay equal attention to cravings. We often crave foods because our bodies are lacking something. If you lack sleep, your body may yearn for quick-energy foods to keep you awake. If you lack love, your body might crave a chocolate bar for that sense of affection and belonging. If your body lacks a certain mineral, it may turn to salty foods in search of it.

What will you learn from your "lab tests"? You'll observe which foods naturally crowd out cravings and give your body the energy boost it needs, then you can introduce those good mood foods into your regular diet. After all, *food is fuel* as well as a source of pleasure. It sustains us, energizes us, and provides nutrients essential to feeling good in both mind and body. Rethink of meals not as simply a source of calories just "to get by" but as the tools to keep our minds emotionally stable and our bodies healthy. Treat your body as a test lab, and you'll see this truth for yourself.

Here's the exciting results of your lab research: eventually, you'll discover that eating nourishing foods helps you overcome food guilt. Higher nutrient-dense foods will help you think more clearly and feel better because they naturally "crowd out" those unhealthy foods that have had you pinned down for years or decades. Eventually, the food guilt will lessen.

Your body is unique. I can't tell you exactly what to eat for your physical and mental equilibrium. I *can* tell you that lots of sugar, additives, caffeine, and white flour make most people feel bad rather than good. I *can* tell you that if you concentrate on adding nourishing foods to your diet, you'll decrease your craving for junk food without feeling deprived.

And it all starts with your awareness and eagerness! Small changes really do add up. The information and recipes in this book are tools to help you move *away from* food guilt and *toward* good health.

3

Master Your Food Moods

Understanding which foods fuel you and your mood can help you shed food guilt sooner than later. Because once you lay the good food mood foundation and feel great both mentally and physically, your body can better combat any stress that comes its way, even if the stress is self-induced from food guilt.

This chapter provides a blueprint for mastering your food moods. It will continue the process of understanding your body's unique needs that we began in the previous chapter. At the same time, it will help release negative food patterns so you can be free from food guilt once and for all.

Foods That Enhance Your Mood

The following chart lists foods that scientists, nutritionists, and health coaches say can lift you up and make you feel energized, focused, sexy, calm, or grounded. Try these foods and see how you feel. Do you notice an energy increase, a decrease, or nothing at all?

Use the third column to list other foods that you've learned produce the desired results.

GOOD MOODS AND REAL FOODS

GOOD MOODS	REAL FOODS TO SUPPORT	*MY* REAL FOODS
Energized	Dark leafy greens Garlic Ginger Lemons	
Focused	Avocados Nuts Quinoa	
Sexy	Asparagus Blueberries Dark chocolate Watermelon	
Calm	Bell peppers Chamomile Coconut water Pumpkin seeds	
Grounded	Beans Beets Carrots Sweet potatoes	

 Food Mood Girl Mantra: While certain foods can boost your mood, no *single* food will be as helpful to your health as consistently eating healthfully. Eating buckets of a superfood like blueberries, for instance, will not counteract a poorly balanced diet! Instead, aim to eat the colors of the rainbow through fruits and vegetables; this can make all the difference in how you feel. Eating a full range of colors each day is an easy way to ensure your body gets the full range of nutrients it needs. Add some protein and grains, and you'll be doing well.

Foods That Deflate Your Mood

Chances are that when you listen to your body carefully, you'll agree with my position that junk foods cause junk moods. I know this not only because of the research but also through my own experience and the experiences of my clients.

The following chart illustrates the most common energy- and mood-deflating foods. When you buy processed or convenience foods, you are more than likely consuming these mood deflators. Pay attention to the ingredient list labels on the foods you currently eat. Are you consuming mood-deflating foods? How does your body react to these widely recognized junk foods?

JUNK FOODS AND JUNK MOODS—AND ALTERNATIVES

JUNK FOODS	EXAMPLES	POSSIBLE JUNK MOODS	QUICK, MORE POSITIVE ALTERNATIVES
White sugar	Refined sugar found in cookies, cakes, and soda; also in health food bars, organic treats	Negative mind-set, foggy thinking, fatigue, anxiety, depression	Natural sweeteners such as honey and stevia
Food additives	Food dyes and colors—additives found in processed and packaged foods—even things you wouldn't expect	ADD, ADHD, negative mind-set, foggy thinking, fatigue, anxiety, depression	Juiced fruits and veggies for color and taste
Caffeine	Coffee, tea, chocolate	ADD, ADHD, negative mind-set, foggy thinking, fatigue, anxiety, depression, acid reflux, osteoporosis	Energizing foods like lemons, dark leafy greens, and ginger
White flour	Typical white breads, cookies, pastries, breading, croutons	Foggy thinking, fatigue, anxiety, depression, upset stomach	Almond flour, brown rice flour, quinoa flour, whole wheat flour

Let's look more closely at these mood-deflating foods and learn how you can swap them out for mood-enhancing, more healthful alternatives.

Good Mood Solutions to Refined Sugar

Imagine a life-size statue of a woman constructed entirely of sugar cubes. That's the amount of sugar the average person eats in one year: 140 pounds. Along with weight issues, many diseases—such as autoimmune diseases, diabetes, anxiety, depression, or even cancer—may stem from consuming large amounts of sugar.

No doubt you know that sugar is a highly addictive substance. Once we eat a little, we want more. It seems like nothing will satisfy our taste buds until we get our next sweet treat. Most people, unfortunately, become sugar addicts without realizing it.

Sugar is hidden in almost every convenience or packaged food we consume, things like granola, health food bars, and even pasta sauces. This makes it difficult to gauge how much we are actually consuming.

So instead of enjoying and savoring a piece of chocolate cake every now and then—without feeling guilt—we end up unknowingly overindulging in sugar daily and experiencing junk moods we can't explain. When we feel junky, we often turn to more junk foods (with their hidden sugars) for "comfort." It's a horrible cycle. No wonder we become addicted!

Have you ever looked at the Nutrition Facts panel on a package only to become confused by the food's high sugar content when nothing in the ingredient list resembles the word "sugar"? This is because sugar goes by names such as corn syrup, sucrose, lactose, fructose, sorbitol, and malitol.

Many of the sneaky sugars you find on a packaged food label are chemically derived and have the same side effects of regular sugar. But at the end of the day, the sugar is still addictive and destructive. The only sugars that work optimally with our bodies are those found in fruit (fructose) and the sweetener derived from the stevia plant.

With that said, I am not suggesting you deprive yourself of the occasional sweet treat, nor am I trying to scare you into feeling more food guilt. Quite the opposite. I believe paying attention to how much sugar you actually eat throughout the day can help you eventually reduce cravings, cut the guilt, and let you fully enjoy the sweet treats you have every now and then.

Awareness is a key to success. I once thought I was being superhealthy by drinking a specific protein shake from a local health food store. One day, I looked at the label on my health drink. Sugar was the main ingredient—at a whopping 32 grams per serving! This was a huge wake-up call. There I was, thinking I was doing the right thing and assuming that every item from a health food store would automatically be healthful. Wrong!

While there is no formal recommendation of how many grams of sugar we are allotted daily, research suggests the lower the better. To new clients beginning to improve their eating habits, I recommend no more than 15 to 20 grams of added sugar per day. We work down from there. "Added sugar" is sugar added during manufacturing to drinks, health bars, and other packaged goods. In contrast, sugar from fruits is healthy, and I tell my clients to eat fruit as often as they want.

Refer to the chart on the next page to start switching out processed table sugar for natural sweeteners. The chart shows how you can use a healthier alternative to replace one cup of refined sugar (table sugar) in baking recipes. As you build success, eventually start improving your recipes by using stevia, which is the only plant-derived natural sugar-free sweetener, in place of other forms of sugar.

REFINED SUGAR ALTERNATIVES AND EQUIVALENTS

Note that formulations and product consistencies are subject to change, but this chart can serve as a quick reference.

NATURAL SWEETENER	PRIMARY USES	TO REPLACE 1 CUP TABLE SUGAR	STEVIA EQUIVALENT
Agave nectar/syrup	Baking, cooking, liquids	¾ cup	¾ teaspoon
Applesauce*	Baking	¾ cup	—
Bananas (ripe)*	Baking	1 cup puree	—
Barley malt syrup	Baking, cooking	1½ cups	1½ teaspoons
Brown rice syrup*	Baking, cooking	1½ cups	1½ teaspoons
Coconut sugar*	Baking	1 cup	1 teaspoon
Dates*	Baking	1 cup puree	—
Date sugar	Baking	1 cup	1 teaspoon
Honey, raw/local*	Baking, cooking, liquids	½ cup	½ teaspoon
Maple syrup*	Baking, cooking, liquids	¾ cup	¾ teaspoon
Molasses	Baking, cooking	½ cup	½ teaspoon
Stevia	Baking, cooking, liquids	1 teaspoon	—
Xylitol	Baking, cooking	1 cup	1 teaspoon
Love*	Anything and everything	Unlimited!	Unlimited!

*Food Mood Girl favorites!

Good Mood Solutions to Food Additives

I took a trip with my mom to a local bed-and-breakfast for a special relaxing weekend. At the time, I had been experimenting with "eating clean" for several months. Eating clean meant eating the way nature intended—lean protein, complex carbohydrates, and healthy fats to keep blood sugar levels stable. I was highly aware of the relationship between the foods I ate and how great I felt.

On the way to the B&B, we stopped at a gas station to fill the car's tank and get some water. As I was about to pay, I grabbed a pack of gum. I popped in a piece of gum.

After two minutes of chewing, I developed a severe headache—the first headache I could remember having in months, maybe even a year.

Why would I suddenly get a headache now? I wondered. Treating my body as a test lab, as we discussed in Chapter 2, I began investigating. Was the headache from the car ride? Was I dehydrated? What did I last eat?

Since I had been eating so well for the past months, the problem had to be an environmental factor. Then I thought about the gum. Examining the package ingredient list, I looked up on my smartphone each ingredient I could not identify or even pronounce.

I was shocked to learn that the yellow #5 (one of the most common food additives) in my gum was derived from coal tar. Yes, tar from the ground. The possible reactions from consuming this substance? Depression, stomachaches, and—you guessed it—headaches.

From that day forward, I decided to respect my body and not give it things like coal tar or other additives. I challenge you to read the labels on your food and look up any ingredients you can't identify. See what is really in your packaged goods. You may be surprised.

Common food additives include:

• Artificial colorings, such as yellow #5 and red #40

• Artificial sweeteners, such as aspartame

• Emulsifiers

• Monosodium glutamate (MSG)

• Nitrates

• Partially hydrogenated vegetable oil

• Pesticides

• Sodium (aka salt)

Given that there are *more than three thousand* food additives approved by the FDA for consumption in the American food supply, additives can quite possibly be making you sick.

Take the time to research what makes up the food you eat. If you see a lengthy list of ingredients, you might want to avoid that food or make a version of it yourself—without the additives. The more you prepare your own food, the more control you have over your health.

Food Mood Girl
Processed Food Guidelines

1. If you can't pronounce it, don't eat it.

2. The fewer the ingredients, the better.

3. If an ingredient has chemical names or numbers beside it, it's probably an additive. It's probably not good for you.

4. Ask yourself, "Would this food taste better if I made it myself?" Unless it's your grandmother's family-favorite apple pie, the answer is almost always yes!

Good Mood Solutions to Caffeine

Caffeine consumption is a frequent topic of debate. While caffeine does confer benefits like alertness and concentration, it also offers its share of problems.

From a food and mood standpoint, caffeine is a naturally occurring drug that can be highly addictive. (Can any of you java junkies relate?) Caffeine addiction can lead to increased levels of anxiety, mood swings, and sugar cravings. Stress levels can actually *increase* while drinking coffee, even though many people believe the beverage calms them down. I've been there.

Check your caffeine consumption daily. If you are drinking too much, try switching gradually to decaf coffee, herbal teas, or Teeccino, which is an herbal, caffeine-free coffee substitute.

The next time your body craves energy, instead of grabbing a cup of joe or a mug of black tea, turn to energizing foods like dark leafy greens, lemons, garlic, ginger, and turmeric. As always, experiment and notice how these foods make you feel. Adjust your intake accordingly.

Caffeine may seem a harmless addition, but addiction of any kind can be harmful. Trust me—I've been addicted to junk food, coffee, alcohol, tea, and kale. Regardless of the type of addiction, the resulting paranoia, guilt, and excessive consumption are no good. It's definitely possible to have too much of a good thing.

Food Mood Girl–Approved Beverages

Green juice

Herbal teas

Lemon water (one-third of a freshly squeezed lemon, or about 1 tablespoon lemon juice, to 8 ounces water)

Teeccino (if you are jonsin' for a coffee)

Turmeric tea

 Food Mood Girl Mantra: Naturally decaffeinate tea by steeping it for three to five minutes in hot water, then pouring out the tea. Add boiling water again to the same teabag. Most of the caffeine will have steeped out in the first brew and you will be left with the flavor.

Good Mood Solutions to White Flour

White flour, white bread, pastas, crackers, cereals, and table sugar: these staples of the American diet typically arrive at their white color via processing or refinement.

Most of these foods are considered "empty" because, during processing or refining, they are stripped of all the nutrient value that their original whole (unprocessed) versions have to offer. Vitamins, minerals, and fiber are lost. The resulting foods are quickly digested, causing us to crave more. Processed foods leave our bodies unsatisfied and craving the nutrients that whole foods provide. In addition, foods stripped of nutrition are quickly converted to sugar in our bodies, causing sugar spikes and drops.

Have you ever experienced the never-ending pasta bowl syndrome? Have you continued eating and eating because you couldn't get full or satisfied? This happens when your body is craving nutrients, not just something to fill the stomach.

Switching from "white foods" isn't necessarily easy if your family relies on convenience foods. The switch is easier when you cook for yourself. Fortunately, the recipes in this book are designed to help you cook at home *without* having to spend excessive time in the kitchen. Recipes like Gram's Pancake Mix (page 47), Happy Quinoa Bowl (page 53), and Connection Cookies (page 114) call for whole grain flours or grains—such as almond flour, brown rice flour, and quinoa flour—that contain the nutrients your body seeks. Most of these flours are available in larger grocery stores.

Food Mood Girl–Approved Flours and Grains

Almond flour

Almond meal

Brown rice bread, such as Udi's Gluten-Free

Brown rice flour

Brown rice pasta

Buckwheat

Quinoa

Quinoa pasta

Rolled oats

Craving-Kicker Station

We touched on cravings several times. Now let's take what you've discovered so far about your own mood foods and apply that to cravings that might otherwise undermine your good nutritional intentions.

It's natural to experience cravings. We humans crave everything we need in one form or another. Cravings happen at different times and for many reasons. They can be hormonal, seasonal, emotional, or biological.

Cravings are the gatekeeper that unlocks the secrets to our unique bodies.

When faced with a strong craving, your first step is to deconstruct it, homing in further with your detective skills. Ask the following questions:

- What do you crave?

- When do you crave it?

- How long have you craved it?

- When did the craving start?

- What is your mood before your craving?

- What is your mood after your craving?

- How satisfied are you when you give into your craving?

- How do you feel after you give into your craving?

Ask yourself these questions regularly. Oftentimes, we crave something but don't stop to determine why. We either give in to our craving and feel bad about it, or we don't give in and continue to struggle with the craving! Answering the questions above will help you understand what you are craving and why.

Once you assess your cravings, use the following chart to take your analysis a step further. Track your cravings for the next week or two in the chart below.

CRAVING TRACKER

DATE	CRAVING	WHEN THE CRAVING BEGAN	MOOD BEFORE THE CRAVING	MOOD AFTER THE CRAVING	OUTSIDE FACTORS (STRESS LEVEL, RELATIONSHIPS, ETC.)

After you track your craving patterns, use the next chart as a guide to further deconstruct your cravings. For example, if you yearn for sweet food, you might want either to cut back on your red meat intake or to work on improving a relationship in your life. Both of these "feed" you in a different way. A need in either area might be causing your sweet tooth.

CRAVING KICKERS

COMMON CRAVINGS	WHAT YOUR BODY MAY REALLY NEED	WHAT TO INCORPORATE	RECIPES
Sweet food	Natural energy Less red meat Detoxifying nutrients Less stress Balance More sleep/rest Quiet meditation Time with friends and family	Dark leafy greens Fish Fruits Sweet vegetables like carrots and sweet potatoes Natural sweeteners like agave nectar or stevia	Connection Cookies (page 114) Chunky Monkey Ice Cream (page 121) Gluten-Free Apple Crisp (page 117)
Salty food	Natural minerals More water	Natural, unrefined sea salt Water and lots of it! Root vegetables like carrots, beets, and potatoes Sea vegetables/seaweed (kelp, kombu, nori, dulse, and others)	Binge-Free Bread Sticks (page 108) Kale Chips (page 107) Brussels Sprouts Chips (page 109)
Chocolate	Magnesium Balance	Raw nuts, seeds, and legumes Fruits Natural sweeteners like agave nectar or stevia Exercise Stress-reducing activities like reading, writing, and yoga	No-Bake Chocolate Pie (page 119) Crunchy Bliss Bites (page 123) Chia Seed Pudding (page 124)
Caffeine	Natural energy Less stress More rest Balance Detoxifying nutrients	Dark leafy greens Raw fruits Raw nuts, seeds, and legumes Whole grains such as brown rice, quinoa, and barley Exercise More sleep/rest	Lemon Tonic (page 100) I'm Berry Sorry Smoothie (page 54) On-the-Go Oats (page 48)

CRAVING KICKERS CONTINUED

COMMON CRAVINGS	WHAT YOUR BODY MAY REALLY NEED	WHAT TO INCORPORATE	RECIPES
Bread/pasta	Whole grains Balance	Brown rice pasta Cauliflower or potatoes Raw nuts, seeds, and legumes Whole grains such as brown rice, quinoa, and barley Time with friends and family	Roasted Cauliflower Mash (page 106) Veggie Bites (page 105) Shame-Free Pizza (page 92)

Refer to this chart whenever you crave a certain food or drink. Feel free to add other foods that you find work for you.

But what if you don't have enough time to whip up one of the recipes listed above? In those cases, I recommend selecting from the following chart of simple snacks. Some of these are perfect to pack and go, giving you the ideal fuel to kick those cravings to the curb—and beyond!

CRAVING-KICKER SIMPLE SNACKS

Keep these quick and easy substitutes on hand to satisfy common cravings and do your body good.

COMMON FOOD CRAVINGS	SIMPLE SNACKS TO KICK THE CRAVING!
Sweet food	1 ounce dark chocolate Apple Banana with almond butter Handful of grapes Sauerkraut Smoothie Sweet veggies like a sweet potato
Salty food	Handful of unsalted or reduced-salt tortilla chips with fresh salsa Olives

COMMON FOOD CRAVINGS	SIMPLE SNACKS TO KICK THE CRAVING!
Chocolate	1 ounce dark chocolate Healthy Hot Chocolate (page 112) Handful of nuts
Caffeine	Fresh fruit Green tea Lemon water
Spicy	Gluten-free or whole grain toast with spicy jam Hot peppers Spicy hummus
Crunchy	Apple Celery with almond butter or hummus Nuts and seeds Popcorn Rice cake Rice crackers
Creamy	Apples and almond butter Avocado Chia Seed Pudding (page 124) Coconut milk Hummus and carrots Soup
Comfort	Small amount of organic cheese on a rice cracker

4

Food Mood Girl Eats . . . Real Food

Many times when I give seminars about food mood and food guilt, curious attendees raise their hands and ask, "So Lindsey, what do you eat on a daily basis?" Or they request my opinion on the latest diet trend.

Let's cut to the chase. The truth is—I don't like labels. In my everyday life, I normally never disclose what I do or don't eat because of the judgments our culture applies to both the diet and the person. People usually assume that because I am a food coach, that means I want them to eat the same things I do. Not necessarily! And then there are those situations where if I'm eating in a way that others disagree with, I often detect a tinge of prejudgment or condemnation in the air. For instance, if you tell vegans that you eat meat, you might have green juice splashed in your face. (And that's only a slight exaggeration!) If you are a vegetarian, people may think you are stuck up or that you eat vegetables for a "diet." If your preferred foods are those from the Paleo diet, people may assume you carry around backpacks full of bricks for exercise and eat nothing but bacon. Of course, most diets have some benefits, and much can be learned from them all. The danger comes when we categorize people based on what they eat and label their approach as "right" or "wrong" or "good" or "bad." Like members of cliques at high school, we can become so focused on what's "in" (in a food sense) that we overlook something of value outside our own usual menu.

All this focus on right and wrong and good and bad translates into anxiety and guilt that sit and simmer within us. Before we know it, we lose touch with our own body's needs because of the assumptions we make based on food fads and societal pressures. It's no different from a concern with clothes, money, or other worldly possessions—oftentimes, we wish to have certain experiences and items because it seems everyone else is doing and owning the same thing. But when it comes to your health, it can be counterproductive or even dangerous to aim to fit in with the status quo. Because your unique body is far from average.

So when people ask what I eat, I reply that I consider myself a "food-mood-itarian." I eat food that I like and that makes me feel good. Most of the time, it's plant based, supplemented with an occasional piece of fish. And about every year or two, I eat a burger of grass-fed beef. I prefer quality foods over diet foods, self-love over guilt. *It's not that I consider my diet to be the answer for everyone. But it works for me.* Ultimately, I want my food to stay true to who I am. And I encourage you to stay true to your own body's needs.

Once you discover the joy that comes along with food, and once you can sit comfortably in your own skin, then you can be freed from the poor food choices that have manipulated your body and your moods for years. From yo-yo dieting to food restrictions to cheat days . . . these can all be solved with one magical ingredient: self-love.

Love is the most nutrient-dense "vitamin" available. No cookie, diet, sandwich, or chip can provide the same nourishment that you'd gain from truly loving yourself, loving your food, and living a guilt-free food life.

Food Mood Girl Real Food Guidelines

When most people open up a cookbook or a recipe book, they immediately wonder, *Okay, what is this author going to make me do? Will I have to give up dairy? Sugar? Meat? Am I eating nothing but fruit? Or am I only drinking a lemonade type of drink for the next fourteen days?*

In this book, I want to be real with you, to tell you what's up about certain food choices that could be affecting your mood and overall well-being. However, the last thing I want is to be arrogant and dictatorial about what you should eat.

Because when it comes down to it, there is no one-size, fail-proof way of eating. Did you know, in fact, that your taste buds change every six months? Your body is constantly evolving. What may sit well with you today might not be ideal five years from now.

That said, for those folks who wonder what I've learned from my research and experience, I share my three important Food Mood Girl Real Food Guidelines:

1. **Eat more real food.** Focus on eating whole and real foods—that is, foods as they come from nature, not things that have been manufactured or highly processed.

2. **Eat more with less guilt.** Yep, you read that right. At the beginning or end of the day, focus on what you can add *more of* to your diet rather than restrict. Eat real food with less guilt and a whole lot more love.

3. **Listen to your body.** This magical machine will tell you exactly what it needs, if you choose to listen.

What about my take on specific food groups? Let's look at how I apply my guidelines to the following foods that nearly everyone has questions about.

Dairy. In the nutrition world, dairy is one of the most controversial topics. That's because some dairy farms inject steroids and the genetically engineered hormone rBGH into their cows to boost milk production, which in turn leads to higher hormone levels in cows' milk. Additionally, many milks, yogurts, and cheeses are pumped with fillers and sugar. Some people get upset stomachs from too much dairy consumption. The human body wasn't designed to process massive amounts of dairy, but dairy products have been a growing staple in Western diets over the last few decades.

Food Mood Girl Guide: If your body can digest dairy properly, then have it as a treat. When choosing dairy, focus on quality. Raw cheeses, cheeses from Europe and Canada (where rBGH is banned), and certified organic, rGBH-free milk are the best choices for people who wish to keep treated dairy off their plate.

Meat. This is another controversial health topic. Some diets call for lots of meat, and others eliminate it altogether.

Food Mood Girl Guide: I believe limiting meat consumption is good for all, mainly because doing so encourages people to eat more fruits and veggies (underconsumed in the American diet!) and to get creative with their protein sources. I also believe you should choose the highest quality meat you can—and choose locally sourced meat, when available. Grass-fed, organic meat is the best. If your farmer loves her animals and treats them humanely, even better. Again, think quality. However, I think this decision ultimately comes down to personal choice based on what your body can handle.

Grains. Whole grain, gluten-free, grain-free, whole wheat, sprouted . . . are you grain confused? Yeah—me, too. Here's the deal. White rice, white flours, and some wheat options have in effect been stripped of their natural bran and of many nutrients, making these processed grains harder to digest and of less nutritional value. Refined white flour and wheat by-products have crept their way into many processed foods, from the obvious (cookies and cakes) to the less expected (like soups, salad dressings, beer, and ice cream).

Food Mood Girl Guide: Whole grains found in their original form—such as brown or black rice, quinoa, millet, and steel-cut oats—are the way nature intended them to be: full of nutrients. For many folks, these are a good dietary starting point. As for gluten-free foods—well, some people need to be gluten-free for health reasons, such as celiac disease or allergies. Other folks feel better when they avoid added gluten, even if they just go without it for a short time.

Not to sound like a broken record, but I truly believe it comes back to you. Your body holds all the answers you need to live a healthy, happy life. You just need to listen to how foods make you feel.

Oils. Fat doesn't make you fat. Healthy fats are good for your body and soul. While there are many oils and fats out there, I suggest staying as real (read: simple and unprocessed) as possible.

Food Mood Girl Guide: For food prepared with no to low heat, use unrefined or extra-virgin olive oil, butter from grass-fed cows, or unrefined coconut oil. For medium-high heats, use unrefined avocado oil or unrefined almond oil. For a bit of sweetness or tang, add sesame oil to your favorite stir-fry or Thai dish.

Salt. Salt intensifies flavor in foods. And our bodies naturally need salt. Does that mean you can set up a virtual salt lick in your kitchen? No. Salt is an important mineral, but we have been conditioned through our consumption of processed foods to take in more salt than necessary.

Food Mood Girl Guide: What matters most with salt is the quality. Choose sea salt, when possible, because it naturally contains more minerals than highly processed table salt—minerals that your body craves. If you notice yourself yearning for salty foods or constantly shaking salt on everything because your food tastes bland, try swapping in other spices to enhance flavor. Fresh herbs and spices can give you a kick and nutrients your body needs without the added sodium.

Sweeteners. Sugar is one of the most common mood deflators, and it is hidden in almost every processed food nowadays.

Food Mood Girl Guide: In all my research, when it comes to sweeteners, the best ones are those found directly in nature, such as coconut sugar, maple syrup, and local or raw honey. See page 19 for the discussion of sugar substitutes.

Make It about You!

Remember, always listen to *your* body, not to the spokesperson of the diet du jour. Follow the results of the "lab tests" you conducted in Chapter 2 and the "blueprint" you drafted in Chapter 3 to eat the foods that energize your body and boost your mood. I'd be surprised if your good foods are not also real foods.

5

Hello, Recipes!

n previous chapters, we looked into the energy you bring to food, the energy food brings to you, and simple ways to take the guilt out of eating. We touched on the Food Mood Girl Real Food Guidelines that work for me and that may work for you.

Now comes the fun part—implementing, cooking, and enjoying!

When it comes down to it, the concept of cooking and eating is simple: *eat real food*. Real foods are the natural, unadulterated foods you find in nature: fruits, vegetables, and whole grains. The human body functions more efficiently with a diet of real food. But don't take my word for it. Eat real food and see how you feel afterward. Compare how you feel when you eat whole foods to your energy and mood after consuming empty, processed calories. Then love your body with the foods that nourish you with good moods.

Recipes with Goals

I created more than seventy recipes with two goals in mind:

1. To heighten your awareness of the emotional elements that surround eating

2. To provide recipes for real food you can make even with a busy schedule

Each recipe shares a guilt-free tip, a short personal story, or an inspiration. And to encourage you to eat and cook with love, each recipe starts with an affirmation. Before, during, and while you are cooking, repeat this affirmation to yourself or out loud. Believe it. Feel it. Create with it. Cook with it. Love it. Savor it. Enjoy it. Most important, embrace it. Carry this newfound energy with you from the cooking process to your plate. Give thanks and savor the taste and love that were poured into your dish.

As you try the recipes, feel free to add your own twists. Adjust ingredients to meet your personal tastes and needs. If you aren't completely satisfied with a recipe, don't give up on it immediately. Tweak the recipe where you can. We are all bioindividually different people, and our recipes should be different, too.

Have fun exploring these delicious dishes as you love your body with good nutrients. Eat well, and remember to provide nonfood nutrients to your mind and spirit, too. You are wonderful. Treat yourself accordingly! Enjoy!

MY CULINARY MUST-HAVES

The following are useful cooking tools. I call them "must-haves" because I can't live without them! They aren't essential, but they are "Food Mood Girl approved" to save you lots of food prep and chopping time.

CULINARY TOOL	BENEFITS	WHERE TO FIND
Cheesecloth	You never know when you'll need a piece! Use this for straining homemade nut milks along with other culinary delights.	Kitchen stores or Amazon.com
Food processor	In a few seconds to minutes, you can process whole foods down to a meal or a liquid. Perfect for making nut flours and butters.	Kitchen stores, Pampered Chef, or Amazon.com
Garlic press	Makes it supereasy to mince garlic.	Kitchen stores, Pampered Chef, or Amazon.com
Glass bowls	Use for mixing, adding to, and storing foods. Plastic bowls often contain BPA and other nasty additives that leach into food; glass does not.	Kitchen stores, Pampered Chef, or Amazon.com

CULINARY TOOL	BENEFITS	WHERE TO FIND
High-performance blender, such as NutriBullet or Vitamix	High-performance blenders excel at preparing soups, dips, smoothies, nut butters, and more. The NutriBullet is ideal for small batches and on-the-go smoothies. The Vitamix is great for family-size smoothies, batches of soups, and nut flours.	Nutribullet.com or Vitamix.com, most kitchen stores, or online
Immersion blender	Easily mix and puree soups or mash potatoes right in the cooking pot. It eliminates the additional mess and cleanup of using a blender.	Kitchen stores or Amazon.com
Mandoline	Whiz through slicing veggies like carrots, potatoes, and cucumbers. Makes veggie platters look unique so that crunching on veggies is fun.	Kitchen stores or Amazon.com
Rice cooker	Make rice in a snap—no more waiting for perfection!	Kitchen stores or Amazon.com
Salad spinner	Wash and dry lettuce, spinach, or any other leafy green quickly and easily.	Kitchen stores or Amazon.com
Vegetable spiralizer	This gadget helps prepare vegetable pasta easily and quickly.	Kitchen stores or Amazon.com

MOOD-BOOSTING SUPERFOODS

These are some of my favorite superfoods that you'll see in the recipes.

MOOD-BOOSTING FOOD	BENEFITS	WHERE TO FIND
Chia seeds	These little seeds are nutrient packed, high in fiber, and a great source of omega-3 fatty acids. Not only do they give you a mental boost but they also make you feel fuller faster so you will be less likely to overeat.	Health food stores, Costco, or online stores like Vitacost.com

MOOD-BOOSTING SUPERFOODS CONTINUED

MOOD-BOOSTING FOOD	BENEFITS	WHERE TO FIND
Nutritional yeast	Nutritional yeast is actually a member of the fungi family. It is an organism found on molasses. It is packed with nutrition, particularly B vitamins, folic acid, selenium, zinc, and protein.	Health food stores, some grocery chains (in the health food section), or online stores like Vitacost.com
Raw cacao powder	Good source of magnesium; tastes like chocolate.	Health food stores or online stores like Vitacost.com
Raw or local honey	Most store-bought honey contains high-fructose corn syrup. Raw and local honey give you the best quality and taste. It also helps some folks with allergies and is a great substitute for sugar.	Local farmers' markets, health food stores, or online stores like Vitacost.com

6

Be-Yourself
Breakfasts

We hear it said all the time: "Breakfast is the most important meal of the day."

A healthy breakfast energizes and prepares you for the hours to come. It nourishes you and makes you feel alive. It's what grounds you and ignites the passion in your bones and the energy to go forward and be your best self.

I look at breakfast as being the entryway not just to health but to being you. Yes, eating breakfast is the most important part of your health routine, but so is getting grounded in who you are.

When dealing with food guilt and emotional eating, I found it hard to accept myself just as I was. I used food to make me feel better or as a tool of self-torment and pain. Being yourself is a lifetime full of work. It's constantly learning about yourself and improving. It's about being able to be okay with where you are in life despite your vision of where you want to go. And it's about looking at yourself in the mirror and smiling at what you see.

As you prepare and eat the morning meal, repeat the recipe affirmations to help let down your walls and discover your amazing gifts. Each breakfast provides a nourishing start physically, but let the affirmations nourish you emotionally.

Be yourself. Take each morning and delve into you.

Be-Yourself Bars

MAKES 12 SERVINGS

♥ **Affirmation:** I fully love and accept myself.

These bars are not only quick and simple to make, but they include some major mood-boosting benefits to boot! With a clear head and a clear heart, you can truly be yourself.

3 cups quick-cooking oats

3 tablespoons chia seeds

½ cup unsalted peanuts, chopped

½ cup semisweet chocolate chips

¾ cup peanut butter, melted

½ cup brown rice syrup

1. In a large bowl, combine the oats, chia seeds, peanuts, and chocolate chips.

2. Slowly stir in the peanut butter and rice syrup. Combine until the mixture forms one large ball.

3. Press the dough into a 9 x 12-inch baking dish. Refrigerate for up to 60 minutes.

4. Cut into 12 squares. Wrap individual bars in plastic wrap or store the bars in a covered container and refrigerate.

Who Knew That "Being Yourself" Could Be So Hard?

For far too long, I tried to be someone else. I was paralyzed by the road society dictated. I felt like I *had* to be the picture-perfect all-American girl, yet I never once stopped to ask myself if that's what I wanted.

So I just pushed along and was swayed by the latest trends, the in crowds, and the number on a scale. I thought possessing certain "things" would give me the sense of self-acceptance or self-worth I was desperately seeking. I attempted to find myself through food, alcohol, clothes, job titles, boyfriends, or whatever else I could cling to that would give me at least a five-minute high.

But as soon as I started coming off my high from the latest fashion or societal trend, panic and fear crept in. And once again, I let my body be a puppet that someone else was directing, telling me how to move, what to say, how to act, what next trend to follow.

From the outside, I looked like I had it all together. But the inside was a different story. I was broken. I was lost. I was everything but the real me.

Sometimes those moments of tragedy—the dark hours of your life, the moments you are so desperately praying to get out of—are the exact moments when you start to find yourself.

And this was the case for me.

After an existential crisis, a battle with food and alcohol, and one final wake-up call, I decided to look inward for the answers I was seeking. I started asking myself the tough questions: Who am I really? What am I meant to do?

Through those questions, I started to shed the mind-set that had been suffocating me for years. I was learning what it was like to finally be me. No strings attached. No pressure from the outside world. I was simply living in my skin.

I sobered up. I loved my body more. I expressed love more openly. I started a mission to help others. I wrote a book. I married my opposite match (a beautiful, tattooed punk rocker). I was able to accept all of who I am. I finally started producing my own life.

I think the expression "be yourself" is more about accepting yourself for who you are. It's not about your actions, it's about a state of being. It's being able to look yourself in the mirror with a heart full of gratitude, letting go of past mistakes that you let define you for far too long and recognizing that it's okay to simply be you.

Embrace who you are without fear of rejection lingering in your mind. Step into your light and feel the freedom that comes along with it.

What are you waiting for?

Type A Smoothie

MAKES 1 SERVING

♥ **Affirmation:** I move through my day with ease.

This smoothie is less about perfectionism and more about the affirmation. Repeating "I move through my day with ease" will help ground you and release any perfectionism you are holding on to. That's why this recipe intentionally mixes up the ingredients a bit! Trust yourself with this smoothie. Don't focus on following the recipe to perfection. Instead, choose ingredients that feel right to you.

3/4–1 cup greens

1/2–3/4 cup berries or 1 banana

1 tablespoon (approximate) almond butter

1/2–1 cup coconut milk or almond milk

Ice cubes

In a blender, combine the greens, fruit, almond butter, coconut or almond milk, and ice until smooth. Enjoy immediately.

I'm a Recovering Type A Perfectionist

I will admit it—I am a recovering type A perfectionist. Yes, I used to pre-plan plans with a side of contingency plans. Perfectionism shackled me. The thought of being late, wrong, or misinformed was enough to send me into a full-out panic—and eating—attack.

I aimed for perfection. I halted my successes. I was always beating myself up for not doing or being enough. This constant rejection of self for even the littlest things left me a broken mess. My first panic attack occurred as a preschooler, so you can imagine how messed up I was by the time I reached adulthood. Yet a part of me always knew that there had to be another way to deal with all these self-proclaimed expectations that were crippling me.

Eventually, after my anxiety attacks and Twix bar overdoses, I found meditation. At first, the thought of meditating engaged my perfectionist behavior.

I would think, *Wait, am I doing this whole meditation thing right? Will I be scolded for not doing it perfectly?*

After much practice, however, I realized that there was no perfect way to meditate and that I had the power to let go of expectations and focus on just being. I let meditation become a habit. I learned to breathe, relax, and go with the flow a lot more.

So—stop right now. Take a deep breath in. Now exhale. Repeat one more time. Doesn't that feel good?

Sometimes, it's just about slowing down and remembering to breathe throughout the day. The more you can make this a practice, the less stress and anxiety you will feel in your life.

Love Me Smoothie

MAKES 1 SERVING

♥ **Affirmation:** I love me for me.

Loving ourselves is a hard thing to do. Sure, we can all say the words. We can pretend we love ourselves. But when it comes down to it, many of us can't find enough room or heart to like ourselves. Starting your day off with a positive affirmation like "I am loved" or "I love me for me" will cultivate the warm sensation of love that is within all of us, even if it is buried deep. So today, think about the things you like and even love about yourself. Hold these close to your heart. Carry that energy into your smoothie.

8 pitted sweet Bing cherries (fresh or frozen)

1 banana

2 tablespoons dark chocolate chips or carob chips

½ cup unsweetened vanilla almond milk

In a blender, combine the cherries, banana, chips, and almond milk. Add ice cubes for a thicker texture, if desired. Serve immediately.

I Am Enough Smoothie

MAKES 1 SERVING

♥ **Affirmation:** I am enough.

Smoothies are a great way to jam-pack ingredients into one meal. You can add fruits, veggies, and nuts. Some days, however, a simple smoothie didn't cut it, and I found myself hungry midmorning. And by hungry, I really mean "hangry":

Lindsey-ism:

Hangry (n): When you are so hungry, you become angry.

This is when I developed the I Am Enough Smoothie. The added oats make this drink more filling and remind me that I lack nothing: I am enough. And guess what? You are enough, too.

½ cup cooked oats

½ cup fresh strawberries

1 banana

½ cup almond milk

In a blender, combine the oats, strawberries, banana, and almond milk. Serve immediately.

what Are You Really Hungry For?

One day I was craving a banana split milkshake. I was ready to hop into my car and drive to the nearest ice-cream shop so I could devour an entire shake myself.

While the intense urge for this banana split milkshake was calling me, I slowed down and asked myself the infamous question that changed the guilt-free food game for me: *What are you really hungry for?*

I realized that while a milkshake would have been awesome to inhale, I was really craving something deeper than a few scoops of vanilla and a banana could supply. I was yearning for the innocence and freedom that I once experienced with food.

As a kid, I could eat a milkshake without a care in the world. I didn't worry about the fat content. I didn't obsess over the calories. And I certainly didn't think a few swallows of it would send my thighs to chunky town (wherever that is).

In fact, the young me never truly cared about the milkshake itself. Sure, it was delicious, and I enjoyed the flavors, but what I savored were the experiences that came with it. Sipping the shake provided an excuse to hang out with friends at night. It was cooling during intense summer heat. It gave me the quality time with my mom I craved.

So next time you have a craving, ask yourself, "What am I really hungry for?" The answer might surprise you.

Banana Split Milkshake

MAKES 1 SERVING

♥ **Affirmation:** I embrace my inner child.

This shake is perfect for those days that you want to embrace yourself by acting like a kid. I suggest drinking it out of a silly straw and laughing so hard that milk comes out your nose. (Okay, maybe not that hard, but you get the point.)

½ cup frozen, unsweetened pineapple chunks

1 frozen banana

⅓ cup Bing cherries

2 tablespoons raw cacao powder

½ cup coconut milk

2 ice cubes

In a blender, combine the pineapple, banana, cherries, cacao, coconut milk, and ice cubes. Serve immediately.

Pumpkin Pie Smoothie

MAKES 1 SERVING

♥ **Affirmation:** I am present to nature around me.

In fall, if you find yourself craving pumpkin pie, here's a healthy recipe to take the edge off!

- 1 peeled banana, frozen
- ½ cup canned pumpkin
- ¾ cup unsweetened almond milk
- 1–2 teaspoons pumpkin pie spice
- 2 teaspoons ground cinnamon
- 1 teaspoon pure vanilla extract
- 1 tablespoon raw or local honey (optional)

In a blender, combine the banana, pumpkin, almond milk, pumpkin pie spice, cinnamon, vanilla, and honey, if using. Serve immediately.

Fall into Pumpkin

Our bodies naturally crave foods that are in season. This is why folks crave strawberries in early summer, greens during spring, pumpkin during fall, and hearty grains during winter.

Our bodies know what we need to be sustained each season.

No matter what season you are in, focus on being present to nature around you and choose to feed yourself with seasonal foods. Appreciate the flavors and unique features each season has to offer.

Gram's Pancake Mix

MAKES 10-12 MINI-PANCAKES

♥ **Affirmation:** I am grateful for my past experiences.

Growing up, I went to my grandma's every Thursday because it was my parents' late night at work. My gram and pap would make my sister and me dinner, and we always got to choose what we wanted. One of my favorite, most-requested meals was "breakfast for dinner," which often featured pancakes.

It's fun to re-create childhood memories through food. If pancakes aren't a sentimental favorite, think of another beloved childhood dish you can re-create with a healthful twist. Doing so honors the memory and feeds you guilt-free.

1½ cups quick-cooking oats

½ cup almond flour

2 teaspoons baking powder

2 teaspoons ground cinnamon

¾ cup almond milk

Coconut oil

1. In a medium bowl, mix the oats, flour, baking powder, and cinnamon. This can be made ahead and stored, covered.

2. When you are ready to prepare the pancakes, add the almond milk and stir until the batter is smooth but not watery.

3. Lightly oil a skillet or griddle and heat over medium-high heat. Ladle batter into the pan and cook for about 4 minutes, or until small bubbles appear and the bottom is lightly browned. Flip the pancakes and cook for about 3 minutes, or until golden brown.

On-the-Go Oats

MAKES 1 SERVING

♥ **Affirmation:** I honor my health and my body.

Since this recipe is prepared in a jar with a lid, it makes the perfect grab-and-go breakfast!

⅓ cup rolled oats

1 tablespoon chia seeds

1 teaspoon ground cinnamon

½ banana, mashed or chopped

1 tablespoon raw or local honey or agave nectar

½ cup almond milk

Dried fruit (optional)

1. In a Mason jar with a tightly fitting lid, stir the oats, chia seeds, and cinnamon. Add the banana, honey or agave, almond milk, and dried fruit, if using. Shake the container.
2. Refrigerate overnight. When you wake up, you will have perfect oatmeal.

Are You Too Busy for Breakfast?

I will admit it—I used to be one of those people who was "too busy" to eat breakfast. I thought coffee and a late lunch or dinner would sustain me through a busy day.

I never looked at food as fuel. I viewed it as a means to an end or an emotional comfort. Once I realized that food was more than just a meal, that it was something that gives us life and that should be enjoyed and appreciated, my perspective changed.

But hey—I am still human. Sometimes I don't have the time to make a gourmet breakfast, and some days I don't have enough time to make a smoothie.

So to solve this problem, I developed the On-the-Go Oats. Make them the night before so you have a quick grab-and-go breakfast ready in the morning. Your time and your health will thank you.

Mini-Breakfast Quiches

MAKES 15 MINI-QUICHES

♥ **Affirmation:** I choose to nourish my body with real food.

One of my infamous mantras is "Eat real food." What is real food?

Lindsey-ism:

Real food (n): You know, the stuff that comes from the ground or grows on trees, not engineered or processed in a lab. Oh yeah, you should also be able to pronounce its ingredients.

Next time you find yourself reaching for those frozen processed meals, challenge yourself to make it better yourself. I bet you can! *And* you can ensure it has *real* ingredients!

Coconut oil

4 eggs

1/2 tablespoon sea salt

1/2 tablespoon ground black pepper

1/4 cup diced onion

1/4 cup diced bell pepper

1. Preheat the oven to 350°F. Lightly coat the cups of a mini-muffin pan with the oil.

2. In a medium bowl, beat the eggs. Stir in the salt and black pepper. Add the onion and bell pepper and mix.

3. Pour into the prepared muffin cups. Bake for 20 to 25 minutes, or until the eggs are fully cooked.

Peanut Butter Raisin Chews

MAKES 12 BARS

♥ **Affirmation:** I fill myself with quality ingredients.

Granola bars used to be a wholesome breakfast food until many companies and brands turned what should be a simple recipe into a contortion of ingredients. Even bars that we assume are healthy may be filled with sugar, food dyes, and food additives—which can lead to depression, dissatisfaction, and extreme hunger.

Say good-bye to store-bought granola bars and make your own with this yummy recipe. They contain but a handful of ingredients, and you don't need to bake them!

> 3 cups quick-cooking oats
>
> ½ cup raisins
>
> 1 tablespoon ground cinnamon
>
> ¾ cup peanut butter, melted
>
> ½ cup raw or local honey, melted

1. In a large bowl, combine the oats, raisins, and cinnamon. Slowly stir in the peanut butter and honey. Mix until the dry ingredients are completely coated.

2. With a tablespoon, scoop out some dough. Form into 1-inch balls and flatten onto an ungreased baking sheet.

3. Refrigerate for up to 60 minutes. Wrap individual chews in plastic wrap or store in a covered container and refrigerate.

Extra-Energy Bars

MAKES 12 BARS

♥ **Affirmation:** I am energized.

Ever experience the midday crash? The one that leaves you *hangering* (see page 44 for a refresher on that Lindsey-ism) for a candy bar or a soda from the vending machine? Oh, have I been there! Here's my solution: homemade energy bars that are perfect for an energizing and sustaining breakfast or that can help you cope with a midday slump.

½ cup raw cashews, chopped

½ cup raw almonds, chopped

½ cup raw peanuts, chopped

½ cup sunflower seeds, chopped

½ cup almond butter or peanut butter, melted

½ cup brown rice syrup or raw or local honey, melted

1. Line an 8-inch square pan with parchment paper or waxed paper.

2. In a medium bowl, combine the cashews, almonds, peanuts, and sunflower seeds. Slowly add the peanut or almond butter and rice syrup or honey. Stir until the mixture forms one solid ball.

3. Press into the prepared pan. Refrigerate for 60 minutes, then cut into 12 squares. Wrap individual bars in plastic wrap or store in a covered container and refrigerate.

Pumpkin Pancakes

MAKES 10–12 MINI-PANCAKES

♥ **Affirmation:** I am present to the world around me.

Growing up, I remember eating microwavable mini-pancakes for breakfast. The sugar rush got the best of me, and I was tired before the school bell even rang. These pumpkin pancakes, however, won't give you the crash that prepackaged cakes will. Instead, they will leave you feeling energized and ready to take on the day!

Olive oil or coconut oil

1½ cups quick-cooking oats

½ cup whole wheat flour or almond flour

2 teaspoons baking powder

2 teaspoons ground cinnamon

1¼ cups almond milk or rice milk

½ cup canned pumpkin

1. Lightly coat a griddle or skillet with the oil. Heat over medium heat.

2. In a medium bowl, mix the oats, flour, baking powder, and cinnamon. Add the almond or rice milk. Stir in the pumpkin.

3. Pour the batter onto the griddle or skillet to form small pancakes. Cook for about 4 minutes, or until small bubbles appear and the bottom is lightly browned. Flip the pancakes and cook for about 3 minutes, or until golden brown.

Happy Quinoa Bowl

MAKES 1 SERVING

♥ **Affirmation:** I am happy.

Quinoa is an amazing mood-boosting food that is not only gluten-free but also an excellent source of protein. Quinoa is extremely versatile, too. You can eat it as a warming breakfast bowl, an energizing cold lunch, or as part of a baked dinner dish. This bowl makes the perfect morning meal to power you up for a full day of being you!

  1/2 cup cooked quinoa (warm)

  1 teaspoon ground cinnamon

  2 tablespoons almond butter

  1/4 cup fresh blueberries

  Raw or local honey

  Almond milk

1. In a small bowl, mix the warm quinoa with the cinnamon and almond butter.
2. Top with the blueberries, then add honey and almond milk to taste.

I'm Berry Sorry Smoothie

MAKES 1 SERVING

♥ **Affirmation:** I choose forgiveness.

Berries contains dopamine, which is a stimulatory neurotransmitter that helps control the brain's reward and pleasure centers. A cup of berries a day is enough to boost your mood and keep you happy!

½ cup strawberries

½ cup blueberries

½ cup raspberries

2 tablespoons raw cacao powder

½ cup almond milk

Handful of ice cubes

In a blender, combine the berries, cacao powder, almond milk, and ice. Serve immediately.

Choosing Forgiveness

Forgiveness is a tough thing. Sometimes, it's easier to forgive people we aren't as close to than it is to forgive the people we love.

Growing up, my parents were always busy, and sometimes it seemed like they were "too busy" for me. As a kid, this caused me an immense amount of anxiety. As I reached adulthood, I realized that these negative seeds were buried deep inside of me and that I let them bloom into weeds for years and years.

These weeds would show up at meals or special events. I would lash out, cop an attitude, or cry my eyes out. I put up these walls and defense mechanisms because I could not understand why my parents were always "too busy" for me.

As my self-awareness rose, I viewed this situation with fresh eyes. And it was then that I discovered the power of forgiveness.

I began to realize that my parents worked hard to provide my sister and me a life they never had. It wasn't that they were ignoring me, it's that they were working *for* me. This eureka shifted my perspective and in turn helped me learn the power of forgiveness.

I eventually understood that Mom and Dad were always doing their best to love me the way they knew how. At the time, it wasn't how I wanted to be loved, but I now realized it was no longer necessary to hold on to resentment and anger.

So I choose forgiveness. While it can often be a tough thing to do, it's necessary for feeling our best and loving others. Forgiveness releases anxieties and helps us gain compassion and understanding for people that we never thought we had.

7

Letting-Go Lunches

The big picture in a healthful life is about letting go, moving through loss or pain, and learning to love yourself and your feelings.

Lunch reminds me a lot of letting go. Lunch usually happens in the middle of the day, and often it can come on quickly. Throughout the day, so much stuff can happen. There can be tension at work, sudden illnesses, annoying e-mails; the list goes on.

So to me, lunch is a perfect metaphor for the time of day to let go and get reenergized. It's a great time to release midday—or midlife!—tension and focus solely on you. The outside distractions can wait. The e-mail will eventually get sent. Let go of the stress and tension and focus on nourishing all of who you are.

Use your lunch to embrace the present moment and emerge with the renewed sense of energy to carry you through the rest of the day.

Granny Smith Grilled Cheese

MAKES 1 SERVING

♥ **Affirmation:** I move through loss with love.

Instead of making the normal white bread, butter, and processed American cheese slices sandwich I was used to, I put a health spin on my version of this comfort-food classic.

1 teaspoon coconut oil

2 slices gluten-free bread

4 mini slices raw Cheddar cheese

6 thin slices Granny Smith apple

1. In a small skillet, melt the oil over medium heat.
2. Place a slice of bread on the skillet. Stack the cheese and apple slices on the bread. Top with the second bread slice.
3. Cook over medium heat for about 5 minutes. Flip the sandwich and cook for another 5 minutes, or until the cheese is melted and the bread is lightly browned.

when a Grilled Cheese made it All Okay

It had been more than a month since my dad passed away. I definitely had been experiencing emotional ups and downs, even though I continued to be grateful for not only what had been shown to me during this time but also the person I had become.

It wasn't long ago when grief have would sent me looking to cookies to make me feel safe or to alcohol to mask the pain. But during this period, I was more aware of my body and myself, and that allowed me to feel more free and relaxed during this grieving process.

That week, however, I was missing my dad more than usual. One night, I got an intense urge for a grilled cheese sandwich. I cannot tell you the last time I ate a grilled cheese, but I can assure you that it had been a while!

You see, when we are looking at food and cravings, sometimes it's a lot deeper than willpower alone. *This craving was all about memories.*

This grilled cheese brought back happy memories of my dad. I recalled all the times he made me grilled cheese as a kid (it was one of my favorites). Dad and I would eat our grilled cheeses together and watch episodes of *Unsolved Mysteries.*

I also remembered the many times after my dad had chemo when a grilled cheese was the only thing he wanted or could stomach. So I would happily make him one (with a side of fresh green juice, of course). It gave me such joy to feed my dad just like he fed me as a kid.

So this grilled cheese craving was no surprise. It brought me great joy to make and eat this humble sandwich—with a healthful twist, naturally. I got to remember my dad and appreciate those memories.

Next time you are craving a specific food, ask yourself if you are really craving a memory instead. If so, respect that memory. Make a healthier version of what you are craving and prepare the food with the love that you feel. It will feed you in a way you have never been fed before.

Cool Beans Salad

♥ **Affirmation:** I am open to all possibilities.

This salad is perfect for a cool summer day. Top a scoop on fresh greens or add some quinoa or brown rice for an added nutritional boost.

1 can (15 ounces) black beans, rinsed and drained

1 red bell pepper, diced

1 green bell pepper, diced

1 cup thinly sliced celery

1/2 cup diced red onions

5 tablespoons olive oil

1/4 cup red wine vinegar

1 teaspoon ground cumin

1/4 cup chopped fresh cilantro

1. In a large bowl, combine the beans, peppers, celery, and onion.

2. In a small bowl, whisk together the oil, vinegar, cumin, and cilantro. Pour over the vegetables and stir until thoroughly coated.

3. Let stand 15 minutes to blend the flavors, or refrigerate up to 2 hours before serving. To serve, spoon the salad onto a bed of lettuce or greens.

Do You Judge Food by Its Cover?

When I was growing up, my dad always used the expression "cool beans." And while I thought the saying was superfunny, the thought of actual beans grossed me out. Even the word "beans" gave me the chills. I vowed never to eat beans in my life! And the funny part is—I had never even tried them.

Have you ever despised a food and didn't know why? Or maybe you tried a food prepared one way and made a snap judgment that it wasn't for you?

I did this with beans. I despised them. I hated them. I couldn't stand the look of them. But I had never tasted them!

Then one day I was forced to eat beans. And after a few bites, I realized that I actually liked them.

Here I was, so disgusted by beans that I never gave myself permission to try them, let alone like them!

When it comes to food, many of our judgments are based on the way a food was prepared or what someone else thought of it. So if you don't like a specific food, ask yourself why. Is it the way it was prepared? Is it the texture? Figure out the reason, and maybe try that food prepared in a different way.

Almond Buddha Bowl

MAKES 1 SERVING

♥ **Affirmation:** I am present in each moment.

Sometimes I don't feel like cooking, but I think I should feel like it. I get so caught up in the *shoulds* and *woulds* that I can't focus on the present moment. Almond Buddha Bowl is my go-to lunch for those times that I don't feel like cooking but still want to nourish myself and enjoy the present moment.

1 banana

3–4 frozen strawberries

1 tablespoon almond butter

½ cup almond milk

1 cup gluten-free granola

1. In a blender or food processor, combine the banana, strawberries, almond butter, and almond milk until smooth.

2. Pour this smoothie mixture over the granola and enjoy!

Listen Up, Butternut

MAKES 6–8 SERVINGS

♥ **Affirmation:** I listen to my body.

There are a million different diet theories with corresponding lists of things you should or shouldn't do when it comes to eating. Instead of getting caught up in countless do's and don'ts, be respectful to yourself by listening to your body. Notice how *you* are feeling, what *you* are craving, and how satisfied *you* are. If you listen closely enough, your body will tell you exactly what it needs.

4 tablespoons olive oil, divided

6–8 carrots, peeled and chopped

1 bunch celery, chopped

1 large white onion, chopped

3 garlic cloves, minced

Sea salt and ground black pepper

2–3 bay leaves

4 cups vegetable broth

1 large butternut squash, peeled, seeded, and cubed

1–2 tablespoons ground cinnamon

1–2 tablespoons rosemary

1. Preheat the oven to 400°F.
2. In a soup pot, sauté the carrots, celery, onion, and garlic in 3 tablespoons of the oil. Add salt and pepper to taste. When the vegetables have browned, add the bay leaves and vegetable broth. Bring to a boil, then reduce to a simmer.
3. Meanwhile, put the squash on a baking pan and coat with the remaining 1 tablespoon oil, cinnamon, and rosemary. Bake for 25 to 30 minutes, or until tender. Place the baking pan on a wire rack until the squash cools slightly.

4. Place the squash in a large blender or food processor and process until creamy.

5. Remove the bay leaves from the soup pot. With a slotted spoon, remove the veggies and add to squash mixture in the blender or food processor. Puree until smooth. Return the squash and vegetables back to the vegetable stock. Taste and adjust seasoning if needed.

Refreshing Spinach and Strawberry Salad

MAKES 3–5 SERVINGS

♥ **Affirmation:** I am amazing.

If you find yourself craving something sweet during the afternoon, try adding fresh fruit to your salads. This will curb sugar craving and give you a natural boost in energy.

5 cups fresh baby spinach

1½ cups strawberries, sliced

½ cup crushed walnuts

3 tablespoons fresh lemon juice

¼ cup olive oil

2 teaspoons raw or local honey

1 bunch fresh basil, finely chopped

1. In a large bowl, combine the spinach, strawberries, and walnuts.

2. In a small bowl, whisk together the lemon juice, oil, honey, and basil. Pour over the salad and enjoy!

Green Gratitude Salad

MAKES 2–4 SERVINGS

♥ **Affirmation:** I am grateful.

When you focus on appreciating your food, think about every step that took the food to your plate. Appreciate everyone, from the farmers who harvested the vegetables to the people who transported them to your local grocery store or farmers' market. Consider the love those involved have for their land and jobs. Think of the person who prepared the meal for you and how much love that person cooked into it. Exercise your imagination! Fast food or farm fresh, think of the same steps. This exercise in appreciation will slow you down, reduce the stress on your body, and nourish you in a positive way.

5 cups fresh baby spinach

1 green bell pepper, chopped

1 cucumber, chopped

2 avocados, diced

¼ cup fresh parsley, chopped

¼ cup olive oil

⅓ cup balsamic vinegar

3 tablespoons fresh lemon juice

Sea salt and ground black pepper

1. In a large bowl, combine the spinach, bell pepper, cucumber, avocados, and parsley.
2. In a small bowl, whisk together the oil, vinegar, lemon juice, and salt and pepper to taste. Pour over the vegetables and stir to mix. Serve immediately.

Savory Slaw

MAKES 1–2 SERVINGS

♥ **Affirmation:** I choose to savor life.

Whenever you eat with friends, take a few minutes halfway through the meal to put your fork down, listen to the conversation, and engage in between bites. Focus on savoring each flavor the food brings to the mix. Appreciate your surroundings and company. Do you notice a difference? Are you fuller faster? Check in with yourself and see what happens!

5 stalks bok choy, chopped

1 Granny Smith apple, sliced

1/2 small red onion, thinly sliced

1/2 cup alfalfa sprouts (optional)

2 tablespoons apple cider vinegar or lemon juice

2 teaspoons raw or local honey or brown rice syrup

1 teaspoon ground coriander

1 teaspoon Dijon mustard

1/4 cup olive oil

1. In a large bowl, combine the bok choy, apple, onion, and sprouts, if using.
2. In a small bowl or shaker container, thoroughly mix the vinegar or lemon juice, honey or rice syrup, coriander, mustard, and oil. Pour over the salad.
3. Serve immediately. If you wish to prepare the dish ahead of the meal, add the apples just before serving to prevent them from browning.

Comfort Lasagna

MAKES 6 SERVINGS

♥ **Affirmation:** I am love.

Sometimes food cravings are all about comfort food. That's because comfort food captures every emotion in a single bite: warmth, smell, heartiness, and memories. Anytime your comfort food craving comes on, try making an updated version of that dish that includes quality ingredients with some fruits or vegetables in the mix. Here's one such example.

   3 cups brown rice noodles, cooked al dente

   1 jar (16 ounces) tomato and basil pasta sauce

   2 cups fresh arugula, divided

   1 cup mozzarella cheese, divided

   2–3 basil leaves

1. Preheat the oven to 350°F.
2. In a medium baking dish, spread 1½ cups of the noodles. Cover them with half of the pasta sauce, 1 cup of the arugula, and ½ cup of the cheese.
3. Repeat the layering sequence, then top with the basil leaves.
4. Bake for 25 minutes, or until the cheese is golden brown.

Simplicity Is Key Salad

MAKES 1–2 SERVINGS

♥ **Affirmation:** I embrace simplicity.

Remember that when it comes to food, less is more! Focus on the quality of the ingredients, not the quantity. When a recipe is simple, you can focus on each of the unique flavors and textures.

   1 avocado, cubed

   1 tomato, chopped

1/4 cup cilantro, chopped

1 1/2 tablespoons fresh lemon juice (about 1/2 lemon)

2 garlic cloves, minced

1 tablespoon olive oil

1/2 teaspoon sea salt

In a medium bowl, mix the avocado, tomato, and cilantro. Add the lemon juice, garlic, oil, and salt. Lightly toss and serve.

Craving-Kicker Smoothie

MAKES 1 SERVING

♥ **Affirmation:** I release negativity and embrace joy.

Greens are the number one food missing from the American diet. By adding more greens to your routine, you will naturally crowd out junk food cravings, increase your energy, and lift depression. Adding greens to smoothies is a great way to incorporate more of these nutrient powerhouses without compromising taste. And while smoothies are typically a breakfast food, it's fun to switch it up and have one for lunch, too! This smoothie is cooling and refreshing, perfect for a hot summer day.

1 cup baby spinach

1/2 banana, peeled

1/2 lemon, peeled and cut into pieces

1/4 cup pineapple pieces

1/2 cup almond milk

Sliver of fresh ginger

Handful of ice cubes

In a blender or food processor, combine the spinach, banana, lemon, pineapple, almond milk, ginger, and ice. Serve immediately.

Much Love Mushroom Soup

MAKES 6–8 SERVINGS

♥ **Affirmation:** I am brave.

It's important to love your food. Go into every encounter you have with food, from preparing to cooking to eating, with a state of love and appreciation. It doesn't matter if you're nibbling on a piece of kale or a piece of cake. Approach food with love, and you'll digest better and stress less.

1/4 cup olive oil

1 medium onion, chopped

2 garlic cloves, minced

4 carrots, peeled and diced

3 celery stalks, diced

1 pound fresh mushrooms, sliced

6 cups vegetable broth

3/4 cups dry barley

Sea salt and ground black pepper

1. In a large saucepan over medium heat, warm the oil. Add the onion and garlic. Cook for 2 to 3 minutes, or until the onion is tender.

2. Add the carrots and celery and cook for 5 to 6 minutes, or until the vegetables are tender. Stir in the mushrooms and continue to cook for 5 to 6 minutes.

3. Pour in the vegetable broth and barley. Stir. Bring to a boil, then cover and reduce the heat. Simmer for about 45 minutes, or until the barley is tender. Add salt and pepper to taste. Serve warm and enjoy!

We Go Together Stir-Fry

MAKES 2–4 SERVINGS

♥ **Affirmation:** We are all connected.

Stir-fries remind me of friendships—you can usually put a lot of different shapes, colors, and flavors in one dish and it goes together perfectly! They are also meant to be enjoyed with the company of others.

Take time to appreciate the people around you and make this dish for loved ones. Remember that your friends and family are a source of nourishment, too!

1–2 tablespoons sesame oil

1 garlic clove, minced

1 small onion, chopped

1 red bell pepper, chopped

2 carrots, peeled and chopped

1 package tempeh, cubed

2–3 cups collard greens

Pinch of sea salt and ground black pepper

1. Lightly coat a large skillet with the oil and heat over medium heat.

2. Add the garlic and onion and cook for 3 to 4 minutes. Add the bell pepper and carrots and cook for 5 to 6 minutes. Add the tempeh and cook for 5 to 6 minutes.

3. Once the vegetables and tempeh are browned, add the collard greens. Cover and cook for 4 to 5 minutes, until the collards are tender. You may need to add a little water to help steam the greens.

4. Sprinkle in a pinch of salt and pepper and toss in the pan. Serve warm.

Grounded Soup

MAKES 8–10 SERVINGS

♥ **Affirmation:** I am grounded.

I've been known to feel out of my head from time to time—in other words, total space cadet. I would stumble on words, forget what was going on, and feel disconnected. It was usually around the time I was eating mainly light fruits and vegetables for days on end. I realized my body was lacking the grounding elements certain foods have to offer.

If you are ever feeling spacey and unable to concentrate, root vegetables might be your solution. Root vegetables provide your body with grounding qualities that can help you think more clearly, concentrate better, and strengthen connections in all areas of your life.

2 tablespoons olive oil

5–6 garlic cloves, minced

1 sweet onion, chopped

5 carrots, chopped

5 celery stalks, chopped

8 cups vegetable broth

3 bay leaves

2 cups wild rice

Sea salt and ground black pepper

1. In a large skillet over medium-low heat, warm the oil and gently cook the garlic and onion, without browning, for 3 for 4 minutes. Add the carrots and celery and cook for 2 to 3 minutes.

2. In a soup pot, add the broth and bay leaves. Transfer the vegetables, then add the wild rice. Bring to a boil, then cover and simmer for 60 minutes, or until the rice is cooked. Season to taste with salt and pepper.

Power Wrap!

MAKES 1 SERVING

♥ **Affirmation:** I am powerful.

One small change can make the difference. Instead of grabbing chips, ask for a piece of fruit. Instead of coffee, switch to water or herbal tea. These small changes can make all the difference in the world. Try making one small swap a day and see how the results add up!

1 gluten-free tortilla

2 tablespoons hummus

Handful of spinach

½ cup leftover bell peppers, carrots, cucumbers, and mushrooms, sliced or chopped

1 tablespoon dried cranberries

1. Lay the tortilla flat on a clean work surface. Spread the hummus over the tortilla. Add the spinach to cover the tortilla.

2. Place the peppers, carrots, cucumbers, and mushrooms in the center and sprinkle with the cranberries. Roll the tortilla and get your wrap on!

Go-To Quinoa Salad

MAKES 6–8 SERVINGS

♥ **Affirmation:** I am magnificent.

This quinoa dish is literally my go-to meal. Anytime I am in a pinch or want to make something that will last me a few days, I prepare this salad. It's nourishing, lasting, and flavorful.

2 cups dry quinoa, rinsed well

1 cup chopped parsley

½ cup chopped scallions

½ cup diced tomato

Additional vegetables, chopped (optional)

¼ cup lime juice

½ cup olive oil

¼ cup red wine vinegar

Sea salt and ground black pepper

1. Cook the quinoa according to package directions. Let cool.

2. In a large bowl, combine the quinoa, parsley, scallion, tomato, and additional vegetables, if using.

3. In a small bowl, whisk together the lime juice, oil, vinegar, and salt and pepper to taste. Pour over the quinoa mixture and stir. Serve on a bed of greens or as a side dish.

8

Grounding, Soul-Satisfying Dinners

inner reminds me of togetherness. It's time for community, for a shared meal. It's the hour to come together and share your day, your hopes, your dreams, and your fears.

It's a time to experiment with new recipes. Some can be great, and some might (alas) suck. Either way, you have the support of the people around you (unless you burn something—then you are on your own. Just kidding!).

Dinner is a great time for reflection. This meal reminds me that it's crucial to have a network of supportive people to help you move through life's challenges and issues. Even if you must eat alone, you can still slow down and express gratitude for the day. Even simple acts of slowing down can make your dinner that much more enjoyable.

Think of dinner as a time to bare all with your community, without feeling judged. Think of it as your safe space for connection and creativity. Let the conversations dance, the emotions release, and the creativity flow.

Bon appétit!

Perception Costa Rican Salad

MAKES 10 SERVINGS

♥ **Affirmation:** I choose to perceive my life with love. I am good enough.

This salad is a staple in my house. It makes enough to feed friends or keep me eating healthfully during a busy week. It's fast, simple, and delicious.

1 cup dry quinoa, rinsed well

½ cup pine nuts

¼ cup olive oil + additional for the skillet

1 tablespoon maple syrup

¼ cup lemon juice

Sea salt and ground black pepper

½ cup diced red bell peppers

½ cup diced red onion

1 bunch parsley, chopped

1 cucumber, diced

½ cup dried cranberries

1. Cook the quinoa according to package directions. Let cool.
2. In a small skillet, toast the pine nuts with a little oil on low heat for 5 to 10 minutes.
3. In a small bowl, whisk together the ¼ cup oil, maple syrup, lemon juice, and salt and black pepper to taste.
4. In a large bowl, combine the quinoa, bell peppers, onion, parsley, cucumber, and cranberries. Top with the pine nuts, then drizzle with the dressing. Toss and enjoy!

A FOOD MOOD GIRL JOURNEY

It was the summer of 2011. I had won a trip with my nutrition school to a Costa Rican resort. Sixty of my peers came together for a week of learning, community, and relaxation in this stunning setting.

I could barely contain myself. Sixty nutrition coaches on a mission! We shared a common bond—the love of good, real food. Can you imagine the kale and raw chocolate we were going to consume this week?

When I arrived at the breathtaking resort, I realized I was probably the youngest person attending the school. This shouldn't have come as a surprise, because I began my health journey at the ripe age of twelve and started my health coaching business at twenty-one. I've always been an old soul of sorts.

One by one, we attendees introduced ourselves and got acquainted on a surface level. We chatted about how we arrived there, described what our businesses were, and selected our goals for the week. I was excited yet unexpectedly nervous.

One evening at dinner, after a long day, I wasn't very hungry. I nonetheless piled a heaping plateful of the vegetarian eats. After all, I couldn't pass up all this homegrown, healthy food, right?

Sitting down at a table of coaches, I began putting fork to mouth. Everyone else was talking about their day and the latest health book, taking a bite or two of food between conversations. But I didn't say a word. I silently and intensely wolfed down my food. After five minutes, I realized that my plate was empty. You heard me—empty, as if it had been washed. It gave "clean eating" a whole new meaning.

Next to me was my friend Laurie. I looked at her plate. She had taken about two bites. I glanced at my colleagues' plates—most were full of food, barely touched.

Shame, anxiety, and embarrassment flooded over me. I thought, *Did anyone just see me gobble my food? I wonder what they are thinking if they look over. Maybe if I get up and quickly grab another plateful, no one will notice that I already devoured an entire serving. Quick—what should I do?!?!? ARGH.*

It's one thing to plow through a meal at home or in a private setting—even in front of close friends, I could probably handle it. But speed-eating a mountain of food in front of health coaches—I was mortified. I should have been enjoying time with my colleagues and savoring my meal, not inhaling it. I was ready to turn myself in to the imaginary food police and confess the sinner's price tenfold.

Why, oh why, would I lose control now? I wanted to cry. Here I was—on a trip I had won to beautiful Costa Rica with sixty amazing health coaches, and yet for the first time in ages, I had been defeated by food.

When the retreat was over, I replayed this moment in my mind often. Six months later, I digested the "why" behind that day I inhaled my food: deep down, I didn't feel good enough, that I wasn't accomplishing enough in my life. Despite the conference's tranquil atmosphere and being amid "my people," I still felt like a stranger in that community. I didn't quite jibe with the health coaches who were a few years older than me, and I seemed more like a daughter to the older ones. So I became nervous and uncomfortable and started using food as my safety net. Instead of focusing on the people and conversations around me and being comfortable in my skin, I chose to hide behind the food by bingeing.

Let me be clear: eating a plateful of food isn't bad! But the reason I ate it so fast and intensely was because I was anxious. I was watching all these beautiful health coaches eat confidently, mindfully, and with love, and yet there I was, feeling out of place and using food as a comfort.

This issue was not new. I struggled with a lingering sense of judgment and criticism from age seven to twenty-one. There, in Costa Rica, this feeling resurfaced even though I had a lot to be proud of and grateful for.

Our overeating and guilt toward food are less about our control over what we are eating and more about our innate sense of who we are. I carried around this "not good enough" baggage for quite some time. Despite eating clean, losing weight, and feeling somewhat accomplished and good about life, I wasn't getting to the core of the issue.

The issue was not the food but my perception of myself. And the answer didn't lie in kale juice, self-help books, or accomplishments *but rather within me.* To truly feel freedom from food, I had to first find freedom with myself.

I needed to choose to see these situations differently. Every time I experienced the sense of "not being good enough," I realized that I had the choice to continue feeling that way or to perceive the emotion in a different manner.

I won't lie. I don't pretend to feel good all the time. I sometimes think of myself as "less than." We all have those days—that's human nature. But I can tell you that since that moment of questioning and digging deeper to understand my relationship with food, I have found an immense sense of freedom.

I no longer blame food. I embrace questioning myself. I enjoy learning about my body and mind. And above all, I choose to perceive myself as good enough.

Do you have a negative mantra floating around your head from time to time? What are you ready to perceive differently in your life?

Sweet Thoughts Quesadilla

MAKES 1 SERVING

♥ Affirmation: I am awesome.

Naturally sweet fruits and veggies are a great way to combat sugar cravings throughout the day, but some cravings are usually less about what you put on your fork and more about what you put in your mind. Focus on nourishing yourself with sweet thoughts today. And remember to tell yourself every once in a while how awesome you are. Because, well, you are!

1 small sweet potato

2 tablespoons coconut oil or olive oil

Pinch of sea salt

1 tablespoon ground cinnamon

1/4 cup cooked black beans

1/4 cup fresh pineapple, cubed

1 gluten-free soft-shell tortilla

1/4 cup almond cheese

1. Preheat the oven to 400°F.

2. Cut the sweet potato into chunks and place on a baking sheet. Lightly coat with the oil, salt, and cinnamon. Bake until tender, about 15 minutes.

3. Meanwhile, in a small skillet, combine the beans and pineapple. Heat for about 5 minutes.

4. In a large skillet, gently heat the tortilla. Top with the sweet potato, beans, pineapple, and nut cheese. Cook over medium heat until the cheese is melted and the tortilla is golden brown.

Finally Full Fattoush Salad

MAKES 2 SERVINGS

♥ **Affirmation:** I am full of life.

Playing with herbs and spices can enhance almost any dish. Yes, even salads! This salad includes the right amount of seasonings to give your taste buds a kick.

1 cucumber, cubed

1 tomato, diced

½ onion, chopped

½ cup fresh parsley, chopped

¼ cup extra-virgin olive oil

4 tablespoons red wine vinegar

2 tablespoons fresh lemon juice

1 small garlic clove, minced

1 teaspoon ground paprika

1 teaspoon ground sumac

Sea salt and ground black pepper

2 cups lettuce or salad greens

1. In a large bowl, combine the cucumber, tomato, onion, and parsley.

2. In a small bowl, whisk together the oil, vinegar, lemon juice, garlic, paprika, and sumac. Pour over the vegetables and lightly toss until the dressing is evenly mixed in. Season to taste with salt and pepper.

3. Serve over the lettuce and enjoy!

Full at Last

I was lunching with my husband, Derek, and our friend one afternoon at this cute little Middle Eastern restaurant. I was excited to try this new Pittsburgh eatery.

I meticulously studied the menu, glancing up and down, trying to figure out what I wanted. Both Derek and our friend settled on the falafel salad. I love falafel, but the fattoush salad sounded especially appealing.

Then food fear and stressful thoughts started kicking in. I muttered to myself, *It's just a salad, I should probably get something else. Maybe I will order some hummus as an appetizer, too. What if I am hungry at the end of the meal? Is this going to be enough food? What if the portion is too small?* The thoughts rambled on and on and on.

When the waitress came to take our orders, I hesitantly ordered the fattoush salad. The second she walked away, I fretted. *I should have chosen something else. I should have ordered that hummus. What if I end up hungry? What if I don't have enough?*

You see, food can tell you a lot about yourself.

In this moment, I was fearful about not having enough. Not being satisfied. Not being full.

We live in a bigger-is-better, biggie-size, overindulging culture. In that moment, I had bought into that fear—a fear of not having enough, of not being satisfied, and of not being full for quite some time.

When my fattoush salad arrived, I was so immersed in great conversation—telling funny jokes and enjoying the meaningful relationships—that my salad became secondary. I ate slowly—not intentionally, but because I was too busy gabbing and laughing half the time to notice.

We paid the check and were about to head out. Then I realized that I was full. That little salad I was so fearful about actually satisfied me. Between the nutrients from the salad and the fulfilling conversation with other people, I realized I was full at last. And the food was secondary.

Positive Patties

MAKES 4–6 BURGERS

♥ **Affirmation:** I am positive.

At the end of the day, it's important to focus on at least one positive accomplishment. If there were things you didn't get done, that's okay, because you can tackle them tomorrow. For now, focus on a success you had. It can be something as small as being on time for meetings or something as big as winning the lotto! Complete the accolades with this health-affirming vegetarian patty.

2 tablespoons olive oil + additional for the pan

½ cup chopped onion

1 clove garlic, minced

1 cup diced or chopped vegetables, such as carrots, celery, mushrooms, spinach, kale, corn, bell peppers

1 can (15 ounces) black beans, rinsed and drained

1 tablespoon sesame oil

Herbs such as oregano, rosemary, or ground cumin, to taste

Sea salt, to taste

½ cup quick-cooking oats

¼ cup cooked quinoa

1 egg

1. In a skillet over medium heat, warm the 2 tablespoons olive oil. Add the onion, garlic, and veggies and cook for 5 to 10 minutes, or until softened. Reserve the skillet.

2. Transfer the vegetables to a blender or food processor. Add the black beans, sesame oil, herbs, and salt and pulse until combined but still chunky. Pulse in the oats, quinoa, and egg. Form the mixture into patties.

3. In the same skillet, adding more oil if necessary, cook the patties over medium heat for 2 to 3 minutes, or until golden brown. Flip and brown the other side.

4. Enjoy on a bun or go topless and add extra veggies!

Awareness Tacos

MAKES 2-4 SERVINGS

♥ **Affirmation:** I am aware.

Are you aware of what you feed your body and your mind? Today, focus on food awareness. Look at each ingredient. Be mindful of how it makes you feel. Raise the awareness of all of your senses. See what you observe.

2 tablespoons olive oil

1 red bell pepper, diced

1 small onion, diced

½ cup fresh cilantro

1 can (15 ounces) black beans, rinsed and drained

2-4 soft corn tortillas

1. Heat the oil in a large skillet. Add the peppers, onions, and cilantro and cook over medium heat for 5 minutes. Add the black beans and cook for 15 minutes.

2. In another skillet, warm the corn tortillas one at a time. Alternatively, warm them wrapped in foil in the oven.

3. Add a scoop of bean mixture to each tortilla and serve immediately.

Clever Kale Pesto

MAKES 2–4 SERVINGS

♥ **Affirmation:** I am clever.

Pesto is typically made with basil, but one day I didn't have basil on hand, only kale. So I decided to give it a go! And I'm happy I did, because this kale pesto is delicious. When it comes to creating recipes, sometimes just a clever twist makes the dish the best!

  2 cups brown rice pasta

  1–1½ cups baby kale

  2–3 garlic cloves

  ½ cup cashews

  2 tablespoons olive oil

  ¼ cup Cheddar cheese or vegan cheese (optional)

  ¼ cup sun-dried tomatoes

1. Cook the pasta according to package directions.
2. Meanwhile, in a blender or food processor, combine the kale, garlic, cashews, oil, and cheese (if using) until the pesto is smooth and creamy.
3. Stir the pesto into the pasta and sprinkle with the sun-dried tomatoes.

Cinnamon Pear Quinoa Salad

MAKES 6–8 SERVINGS

♥ **Affirmation:** I am excited by life.

Always aim for healthy. We Americans have a crazy phenomenon where we think "skinny = healthy." Remember that yours is a unique body. Embrace your features and your curves. Focus on being *healthy*, and that will carry you far. After all, good health is your sexiest feature.

Note that this recipe's dressing is a minimalist version. You may wish to add more oil or vinegar, depending on your taste.

2 cups dry quinoa, rinsed well

1/4 cup olive oil

3/4 cup pear balsamic vinegar

1 tablespoon ground cinnamon

Sea salt and ground black pepper

2 pears, cubed

1 cucumber, cubed

1/2 red onion, chopped

1/2 cup unsweetened dried cranberries

1. Cook the quinoa according to package directions. Let cool in the refrigerator.

2. In a small bowl, whisk together the oil, vinegar, cinnamon, and salt and pepper to taste. Set aside.

3. Once the quinoa has cooled, stir in the pears, cucumber, onion, and dried cranberries. Slowly pour the dressing over the quinoa mixture and incorporate evenly through the salad. Add more oil or vinegar, if desired.

Cozy Quinoa Casserole

MAKES 6–8 SERVINGS

♥ **Affirmation:** I am willing to ask for help.

As you make this dish, think of its ingredients like the people in your life. You need people to make life delicious. You need people to help make something good even better.

Make this tasty casserole even more visually satisfying by using tricolor quinoa.

1½ cups dry quinoa, rinsed well

3 cups vegetable broth

1 can (15 ounces) black beans, rinsed and drained

1 tablespoon ground cumin

1 large sweet potato, peeled and cubed

1 red bell pepper, chopped in large pieces

½ red onion, chopped

2 tablespoons olive oil

Sea salt and ground black pepper

1. Preheat the oven to 450°F.

2. Cook the quinoa according to package directions, but use the vegetable broth instead of water. Once the quinoa has cooked, remove from the heat. Add the black beans and cumin. Cover and set aside.

3. Meanwhile, in a medium bowl, toss the sweet potato, bell pepper, and onion with the oil. Add salt and pepper to taste. Place the vegetables in a casserole dish and bake for 25 minutes, or until the sweet potatoes are tender. Stir in the quinoa mixture and serve.

A FOOD MOOD GIRL JOURNEY

I am strong, resilient, and usually appear to have my stuff together.

In the past three years, I've accomplished a lot. I published three books, quit my full-time job to pursue my dreams, rapped onstage for the first time, became engaged, got married, and bought a house. I think I completed every major life event except having a child. (Don't expect that anytime soon!)

While on the outside it seemed like things were going well, and I appeared to have my life all together, the behind-the-scenes view of the past three years have been quite difficult. (I am human, after all!)

With the achievements came dramatic change, lots of uncertainty, and an overwhelming sense of loss. In one year, I lost three uncles, a friend from high school, and my childhood dog—and then my dad passed away from cancer.

I attempted to handle these losses with grace and poise. A week after my dad died, I gave a keynote address about leadership to a group of college students at Carlow University. Despite all the personal upheaval, I still hustled and stayed busy. I would show up and do my thing, without ever feeling sorry for myself or being upset with what had happened.

Of course, I would break down and cry every now and then, but hey, that's just surface-level, normal stuff that happens during grieving, right?

What I didn't realize was that I had been slowly, quietly slipping into a depression.

Let me explain.

Derek and I purchased a house just a few weeks after we got hitched. While it was an exciting time, it was also intense. We had to be out of our apartment and into our new house within two weeks. In those fourteen days, we needed to refinish the hardwood floors, give the house a paint job, and tile the kitchen floor. We were on a major time crunch.

During this period, I started coming off my self-induced high and finally experienced the intense emotions of sadness, loss, and grief.

You see, my dad had been a carpenter and owned a flooring business. I found myself grieving or getting angry with each decision I had to make. Every time I had to choose a color or finish, I kept thinking, "If only my dad was here, he would give me the best advice. He would help make this house the best it could be."

Watching our hardwood floors get refinished made me miss my dad fiercely. Ray, our go-to floor refinisher, was a good friend of my dad's. As he worked, Ray shared uplifting and funny stories about him. While I thoroughly enjoyed hearing the tales, I eventually lost my grip. It was too much. The depression and grief that I had tried to push aside came crashing down on me, and I just sat on my front porch and sobbed with Ray. I told him about my grief and how I'm not perfect and how I need help and support in dealing with everything from the floors to my feelings.

I found myself sinking deeper and deeper. Once Derek and I were moved in and somewhat settled, I began disconnecting myself from projects, people, and anything that felt remotely of a drain. I dismissed things that once gave me satisfaction and great joy. I stopped answering phone calls (even from really good friends). I was unable to take on new clients. I couldn't get excited for friends getting married or going through positive change.

Physically, I was unable to function fully. I would wake up and sit at my computer for hours, unable to focus on anything for more than a minute. A simple task would take days or weeks to accomplish. I beat myself up for not being able to achieve more. Yet I was afraid to ask for help. I put on my social media game face and Instagramed a photo of my kale smoothie like nothing was different. *But underneath it all, I had changed.* I was not the same person I was a year or two ago. I had undergone an intense few years, and who I am as a person evolved because of it.

Ultimately, I realized that no matter what the situation or how spiritual, enlightened, or inspirational each of us may be, we all need help at different times in our life.

And it's important to ask for it when we need it most.

I think of help just like I think of a casserole. All the ingredients work together and complement each other to make it delicious.

We need help in our lives to deal with unexpected tragedies, a task we can't possibly do on our own. Sometimes we just need a listening ear. Remember that it's okay to ask for help when you need it most.

Collard Greens Fajita Wraps

MAKES 2 SERVINGS

♥ **Affirmation:** I make fun a priority!

Don't let the greens fool you. These fajita wraps are not only delicious but also gluten-free and a unique way to ensure you get your greens! The hot ingredients steam inside the wrap so that the collards are crisp and fresh but easy to chew. Unlike tortilla shells, collards don't break apart on you, making them a mess-free dish. Did I mention collards also save you the calories that tortilla shells add on? A win-win for both taste and health!

½ teaspoon cayenne pepper (or more, if you like heat)

2 teaspoons ground black pepper

2 teaspoons sea salt

2 teaspoons ground paprika

1 teaspoon garlic powder

1 tablespoon coconut oil

3 garlic cloves, minced

1 large onion, chopped

1 red bell pepper, chopped

2 collard leaves, de-stemmed and torn into tortilla-size pieces

1. In a small bowl, mix the cayenne pepper, black pepper, salt, paprika, and garlic powder to make the fajita seasoning.

2. In a large skillet, heat the oil. Add the garlic and cook for 2 minutes. Add the onion and bell pepper and cook for 3 to 4 minutes. Stir in the fajita seasoning. Cook for an additional 5 to 7 minutes, or until tender.

3. Spread a collard leaf open on a plate. Top with half of the seasoned vegetables. Repeat with the other leaf.

4. Add any additional toppings such as your choice of meat, hot sauce, guacamole, salsa, cheese, and lettuce, if desired. Wrap like a tortilla shell and serve immediately.

Spiritual Stuffed Peppers

MAKES 4 SERVINGS

♥ **Affirmation:** I step into the light of who I am.

Food is a spiritual journey. There are ups and downs. There are "advocates" and "guides" to help you. However, the spiritual journey is about becoming the best version of you.

As you eat more nourishing foods, your mind becomes clearer. Your body becomes healthier. You are suddenly more open to possibilities and passions than you ever were. You feel better than ever. You are nicer, kinder, and more outgoing. You have the confidence to do the things you've been talking about for years but had never acted on.

You find yourself.

And it all started by choosing to eat foods that lift you up, give you life, and show you who you really are.

1 small + 4 large green bell peppers

1 tablespoon olive oil

3 garlic cloves, crushed

1 onion, chopped

1½ cups cooked quinoa

1 can (16 ounces) stewed or chunk tomatoes

1 can (15 ounces) chickpeas, rinsed and drained

Sea salt and ground black pepper

1. Preheat the oven to 350°F.

2. Cut off the tops of the bell peppers. Scoop out the seeds and pithy membrane, taking care not to puncture the skin. Set the hollowed-out peppers aside. Chop the small bell pepper and the large pepper tops, discarding the stems.

3. Heat the oil in a large skillet over medium heat. Add the chopped bell pepper, garlic, and onion and cook for about 3 minutes, or until softened. Remove from the heat and mix in the quinoa, tomatoes, and chickpeas.

4. Fill the bell peppers with the quinoa mixture. Place them upright in an oven pan or casserole dish. Pour ½ inch of water into the pan to help them steam, cover, and bake for 45 minutes, or until the peppers are soft. Add salt and black pepper to taste.

Funny Fried Rice

MAKES 4–6 SERVINGS

♥ **Affirmation:** I am funny.

Laughter is good medicine. Put on a funny video, think of a funny time, and laugh while you cook! The good energy will carry you through the night.

1 small onion, chopped

1 tablespoon olive oil

2 garlic cloves, minced

1 carrot, diced

½ bunch scallion, chopped

1 tablespoon ginger, grated

4 cups cooked long-grain brown rice

2 tablespoons tamari soy sauce

1 teaspoon toasted sesame oil

2 eggs

1. In a large skillet, cook the onion in the oil for 5 minutes. Add the garlic and carrot and cook for 4 minutes. Add the scallion and ginger and cook for about 4 more minutes.
2. Add the rice, sprinkling it with a bit of water to help steam the dish. Mix in the soy sauce and sesame oil.
3. Crack the eggs and scramble into the mixture in the skillet. Lower the heat and cook for 5 minutes, stirring occasionally. Serve immediately.

Spaghetti Already?

MAKES 2 SERVINGS

♥ **Affirmation:** I am courageous.

Spaghetti was a staple meal in my family's house. It was quick, easy, and didn't take much thought to put together. However, it usually left me overstuffed, anxious, and tired.

As I got older, I tried finding new ways to experience spaghetti without the crash later on. Then I discovered the aptly named spaghetti squash! This squash has the look and feel of spaghetti with all the veggie-goodness nutrients intact. And it won't leave you feeling groggy, tired, or anxious!

Olive oil

1 spaghetti squash

½ cup marinara sauce

"Parmesan" Nut Cheese

½ cup crushed walnuts

¼ cup nutritional yeast

½ tablespoon sea salt

1. Preheat the oven to 375°F. Coat a large baking sheet with the oil.
2. Slice the squash in half lengthwise. Using a large spoon, scoop out the seeds and discard. Place each squash half skin side up on the prepared baking sheet. Bake for 45 minutes. Flip the squash and bake for 15 minutes. Remove from the oven and let cool for 5 minutes. Then, using a fork, scrape out the strings of squash and place in large bowl.
3. Heat the marinara sauce in a small saucepan.
4. Meanwhile, make the "Parmesan" nut cheese: in a blender or food processor, pulse the walnuts, nutritional yeast, and salt until a grainy mixture forms.
5. Stir the marinara into the squash. Top with the nut cheese and serve.

Peary Good Salad

MAKES 4–6 SERVINGS

♥ **Affirmation:** I am bright.

This salad can brighten up any table. It's sweet, savory, and refreshing—perfect for a hot summer day.

½ cup walnut halves

4–6 cups arugula

1 pear, chopped

3 tablespoons fresh lemon juice (1 lemon)

3 tablespoons extra-virgin olive oil

Sea salt, to taste

Freshly ground black pepper, to taste

1. In a small, dry pan over medium heat, toast the nuts, stirring frequently, until lightly toasted. Watch carefully so they don't burn. Let cool.

2. Combine the arugula and pear in a salad bowl, then add the nuts.

3. Add the lemon juice and oil, and season to taste with salt and pepper. Stir to mix, then serve.

My Road to Peary Good Salad

I decided to become a vegetarian for health reasons, because I knew my SAD (standard American diet) eating habits were not doing much for me. But here was the hitch: I didn't like most vegetables and fruits. I could stomach apples and maybe some green beans, but that was pretty much it.

The first month, I honestly didn't know what to eat, so my diet consisted of nothing but brown rice and broccoli. Then I bought and tried any and every product that was labeled "vegetarian." Eventually, I realized that I was becoming a SAD vegetarian: I was eating mainly processed food. The only real food I consumed was broccoli.

Then I decided to shake things up by eating foods out of my comfort zone. Every week, I tried one different fruit or vegetable prepared in different ways and figured out which way I liked it best. Over time, I started loving and appreciating my food for all the vast flavors, textures, and creativity I could get with my new lifestyle.

So I encourage you to try one new food a week and see how you like it. Do you prefer it grilled, steamed, baked, sautéed, or raw? Is it pleasing hot, cold, or mixed in with other ingredients?

The more you experiment, the more you will understand your unique tastes. And you might just uncover new favorite foods!

Shame-Free Pizza

MAKES 4–6 SERVINGS

♥ **Affirmation:** I honor my food choices.

Pizza was a staple in our house when I was a kid, and I'd be lying to say that I don't love it! However, I noticed that the more I got into health, the more pizza became a shaming food for me. It was something that I would get extremely anxious about, and as a result I cut it out of my life for a little bit. Eventually I found a healthy balance and started experimenting with fun and different types of pizza. This recipe is one of my favorites. I also enjoy a slice from the local pizza joint, too!

Olive oil or coconut oil

1 small or ½ large cauliflower

2 organic eggs

1½ cups mozzarella cheese or vegan cheese, divided

4 tablespoons Italian seasoning

Pinch of sea salt and ground black pepper

1 jar (12 ounces) pizza sauce

Veggies of your choice

1. Preheat the oven to 350°F. Lightly coat a baking sheet with oil.

2. Using a box grater or a food processor, grate the cauliflower.

3. In a large bowl, combine the cauliflower, eggs, ½ cup of the cheese, Italian seasoning, and salt and pepper. Mix thoroughly.

4. Spread the mixture evenly on the prepared baking sheet. Bake for about 30 minutes.

5. Remove from the oven. Spread on the sauce, remaining cheese, and vegetables and bake for another 10 to 12 minutes, or until the cheese is melted. Let cool for 5 minutes, then serve.

It's Pizza Time!

Ahhh, pizza! I love pizza. It's probably one of the best culinary inventions to date. Pizza encompasses all my favorite foods into one delicious bite. Just the simple smell of a freshly baked pie is enough to send me into a state of pure bliss.

At one point, though, pizza was my weakness. Anytime I tried a new fad diet, the food I really wanted to cheat with on the diet was pizza. It was the one food I felt like I could never give up, and I would shame myself for hours over a single slice.

I always labeled pizza as "bad" and "no good." I used it as a punishment. It became a torture tool. And it became the worst food humanly possible to eat.

I remember hanging out at a friend's house, and they would order a pizza with lots of veggies for everyone to enjoy. I would pick off and eat the veggies and smell the rest of pizza, thinking that would be enough to get me through the evening.

Other times, I would give in to temptation and eat a single bite. I felt like one big bucket of shame. *Even one bite* made me feel like a loser. It didn't help that my head was slurring profanities at me like, *Lindsey, you suck. Why the #%$@ would you take that bite? You're an idiot. You suck. You are the worst at diets. You are going to die.*

No wonder that immediately after one bite I felt bloated, fat, and 10 pounds heavier. I also felt sick, upset, and unable to experience any joy around me. And this was all from a bite of pizza!

Why did food have so much control? It had the power to take me from happy to sad in literally a single bite.

Then I realized it wasn't the food. It was me. I let pizza have control of me: I had allowed myself to feel shame, anxiety, and guilt whenever I was around pizza. I was so preoccupied with shaming myself over eating pizza that I was unable to enjoy the time with my friends and family or to nourish myself positively. Once I understood that I had control over food, that I had the power to enjoy pizza or anything else in moderation, I could finally attend food functions and not obsess about whether what I ate was "good" or "bad." I could savor an ooey-gooey slice and have fun with my friends without torturing myself mentally.

So if you are going to eat pizza, regardless if it's my cauliflower creation or an XL pie from a local pizzeria, release the tension and anxiety and focus on slowly savoring every bite. Your stomach and your head will thank you.

Embracing Quiche

MAKES 4–6 SERVINGS

♥ Affirmation: I embrace the present moment.

Quiches are my go-to dish when I don't feel like doing much cooking. They are filling, feed several people, and can be designed around whatever vegetables you have in your fridge. It's a perfect way to use up those extra bits of veggies left over from another recipe.

1–2 potatoes, peeled and thinly sliced

1 tablespoon coconut oil + additional for pan

1/2 onion, diced

1/2 cup kale

5 eggs, beaten

1/4 cup sun-dried tomatoes

1/4 cup feta cheese

Pinch of sea salt

1/2 tablespoon ground black pepper

1. Preheat the oven to 400°F. Lightly coat a glass pie pan with oil.

2. Layer the potato slices on the bottom and sides of the pan to form a crust. Set aside.

3. In a large skillet, melt 1 tablespoon coconut oil. Add the onion and kale and cook for 5 to 10 minutes.

4. Transfer the onion and kale to a large bowl. Add the eggs, sun-dried tomatoes, feta, salt, and pepper and combine. Slowly transfer to the prepared pan. If desired, top with additional cheese or sun-dried tomatoes. Bake for 30 minutes, or until the eggs are fully cooked.

Embrace the moment

Have you ever driven to a destination and, on arriving, couldn't remember exactly how you got there? Have you ever looked at your finished plate, not remembering what you just ate?

We are so focused on our fast-paced lives that we often forget to pay attention to life's remarkable details. Without blinking an eye, we rush by signs, nature, houses, and people.

Tonight, focus on being present with your food and your company. Really listen to what people are saying. Experience all the flavors that life and your food have to offer.

9

Sides, Snacks, and Safe Splurges

S nacks, sides, and splurges are great reminders of the extras in life that make it fun and exciting. They can satisfy a craving, provide us with extra nourishment, and hold us over until the next meal.

In life, it's important to get nourishment from the extras that make you feel good. Maybe it's going on a weekend trip, getting a massage, or spending the day writing. These extras—whether they include food or not—give us a sense of energy, renewal, and satisfaction that can carry forward for hours.

Enjoy these recipes and view the dishes as happy "extras" in life. Reach for them when you are feeling hungry or need an added boost in your day.

Hangry-Free Bites

MAKES 12–16 SERVINGS

♥ Affirmation: I am satisfied.

Freeze these bites to salve a late-night sweet craving without the guilt!

½ cup cashews

¼ cup coconut shreds

¾ cup quick-cooking oats

1 teaspoon sea salt

2 tablespoons raw cacao powder

6 teaspoons coconut oil

2 teaspoons raw or local honey

½ cup almond butter

1. In a blender or food processor, pulse the cashews and coconut until finely ground. For a little crunch, process a little less.

2. Transfer the mixture to a medium bowl and add the oats, salt and cacao. Stir. Add the oil and mix well. Gradually stir in the honey and almond butter until the mixture forms a ball.

3. Scoop the mixture by teaspoonful and roll into 12 to 16 balls. Store in an airtight container in the refrigerator for up to a week.

Are You So Hungry You Become Angry?

Empty stomach. Hungry. Full of rage, tears, or sheer panic.

You think, *I need to eat. If I don't eat in the next five minutes, I am going to explode!*

Suddenly, everything and everyone around you are annoying. You flip out for no reason. You scream uncontrollably. The misinterpretation of a tweet from a famous celeb makes you burst into tears. (Yes, hunger can make you be that dramatic.)

Finally, you get your hands on some food. You want it all for yourself. You wonder if it will be enough to satisfy the deep, lingering hunger pains.

You dive in headfirst. As you take a few bites, you loosen up a bit. You feel the food entering your system, and you start feeling somewhat normal. As you finish your meal, a sense of euphoria descends. You're happy, peaceful, and full of bliss.

You apologize to those around you for being so angry and upset just moments earlier. You don't know what just came over you, but you are glad it passed.

This is what I call "hangry." Yes, it is an actual phenomenon. I made up the name, but the feeling is real.

Hangry is when you are so hungry that you become extremely angry, anxious, or even depressed. You may act out, name call, and go into an extreme rage.

Before I studied the link between food and mood, I thought this type of behavior was normal. I would have these attacks at least once a day and would blame it on drops in blood sugar, PMS, or other problems in my life.

But I soon realized that being hangry was a lot more internal than I thought. Ninety-five percent of stress hormones sit in the gut, and so hunger pains affect a lot more than just your hunger level. They can affect your attitude as well.

Being hungry causes serotonin levels to drop, which can lead to withdrawal-like symptoms such as anxiety, stress, anger, and sadness.

After many episodes of hanger, I realized I needed to have something fast and easy on hand to tame my hangry-self. Let's face it—I didn't want to get arrested for cussing out a neighbor or crying in the middle of the produce aisle at Whole Foods. (Seriously, I would get that hangry.)

So I developed my recipe for Hangry-Free Bites to call on in case of an emergency. They are sweet, salty, and packed with protein to satisfy any craving or mood!

My Mocktail No. 1: Lemon Tonic

MAKES 1 SERVING

♥ **Affirmation:** I honor my body and everything that I put in it.

Spicing up your drinks can be fun and refreshing, especially if you don't drink alcohol or just want something instead of water. The lemon tonic is my favorite go-to drink. Not only are lemons great for your health and provide detoxifying benefits, but having this variation truly makes you feel like you are drinking a cocktail.

  1 cup sparkling water

  1½ tablespoons fresh lemon juice (½ lemon)

  Handful of ice cubes

In a shaker or tall glass, shake or stir together the water, lemon juice, and ice. Serve immediately.

My Mocktail No. 2: Minty Fauxjito

MAKES 1 SERVING

♥ **Affirmation:** I release all negativity from my life.

I will admit, mojitos were one of my favorite alcohol-based drinks. So this mocktail is a sweet and minty version minus the booze but adding all the energizing benefits of the natural ingredients.

  ½ cup fresh kale

  1 banana

  Handful of fresh mint

  ½ lime, peeled

  Handful of ice cubes

In a blender or food processor, add the kale, banana, mint, lime, and ice. Process until smooth and serve immediately.

A FOOD MOOD GIRL JOURNEY

There was a point postcollege and pre–health coach career where I was slowly making my way into mainstream living. Just days before my twenty-second birthday, I had a full-time job, I was getting my health back on track, and I was six months into my training program at nutrition school. I was also building my business and working on my first book.

Although I was now super into eating healthy, I still struggled with my new identity. I went from latte loving to kale smoothie drinking; from thinking that being stressed was awesome to meditating; from a career in public relations to a career in nutrition. Needless to say, I was having a bit of an identity crisis.

But I was afraid to face a bigger demon that had haunted me for years. I was a closeted emotional alcoholic.

I describe an emotional alcoholic as one who binges on alcohol and uses it as a crutch to mask true feelings. They don't need to drink every day. But when they do drink, no stop is in sight.

I convinced myself that if I consumed enough kale juice, it would outweigh my vodka binges. "Well, I can get blackout drunk tonight, and tomorrow I can drink wheat grass shots to detox." The sad thing was, I seriously believed that crazy theory.

Then my twenty-second birthday arrived.

I was excited to gather my friends and my mom together for a vodka-filled celebration. We planned to attend a concert that evening. Everyone arrived at my apartment around 4:00, and we started drinking shortly after.

A cab was on its way, and I remember thinking, *I'm not drunk enough to go to this concert.* In my mind, in order to have fun and feel good, I had to be heavily buzzed. So as the cab pulled up, I pretended to forget something upstairs. Everyone else headed to the cab; I raced to my closet. I pulled out a bottle of vodka and chugged.

I vaguely remember walking back downstairs and stepping into the cab. Then everything went blank.

I only know what happened next because my mom and friends told me. Apparently, when we arrived at the stadium, I was swirling and slurring words. People walking by stared and pointed at me. My friends videoed me with their phones.

Just as I passed out on the concrete slab, a cop came over to my mom and asked, "Um, is she okay?"

"She is sick, and I am taking her home right now," my mom immediately replied.

Mom was right. I was sick. I had a problem. And I needed major help.

I woke up fourteen hours after my vodka coma alone in my bedroom with a glass of water on the nightstand. I felt ashamed and remorseful. *What the heck happened?* I wondered. I had no recollection of the night after leaving my apartment.

Suddenly an inner voice said, "Lindsey, your purpose in life is far greater than alcohol will ever be. Get sober, and good things will come."

In that moment, I realized I was jeopardizing my health, my happiness, my career, and my spiritual path by letting a substance control me. From that day on, I committed myself to sobering up and getting comfortable with being uncomfortable as I transitioned.

I removed myself from the bar scene and got rid of alcohol paraphernalia in my house. I lost friends and felt alone, ashamed, helpless, and as if I wasn't fun anymore. Many people didn't understand why I quit, and some still don't. Because I didn't crave alcohol every day, they didn't think I had a problem. But you don't have to drink alcohol day and night to have a problem with alcohol. You just have to drink it for the wrong reasons.

I recognized that my emotional eating habits were no different from my emotional drinking ones. To mask insecurities and shame, I had just switched substances. But no kale smoothie could combat my addiction to vodka.

I haven't had alcohol since that birthday. Now I embrace my new way of living and have made *not* drinking kind of cool. I switched vodka and sodas for my Lemon Tonic and traded up my mojitos for a Minty Fauxjito.

Pumpkin Hummus

MAKES 6–8 SERVINGS

♥ **Affirmation:** I am creative.

This pumpkin hummus is the perfect example of how I let my taste buds and creativity guide my cooking experiments. I put love, creativity, and passion into this recipe, and I hope you do the same! Note: This hummus goes great with cinnamon pita bread or plain rice crackers.

1 can (15 ounces) chickpeas, rinsed and drained

7½ ounces pumpkin puree (from a 15-ounce can)

2 tablespoons tahini

2 tablespoons raw or local honey

1 tablespoon pumpkin pie spice

¼ teaspoon sea salt

1–2 tablespoons water, divided

1. In a blender or food processor, combine the chickpeas, pumpkin, tahini, honey, pumpkin pie spice, salt, and 1 tablespoon of the water until smooth and creamy, pausing occasionally to scrape the inside of the bowl with a spatula. If the mixture is too thick, add another tablespoon of water.

2. Refrigerate for 2 hours in an airtight container before serving.

Find Your Inner Chef

I wasn't born a culinary expert. The only thing I could prepare for a very long time was a low-calorie frozen meal or a salad.

But I started experimenting in the kitchen and let go of expectations. If a dish turned out to be a masterpiece—great! If it was just "okay," that was fine, too! I focused on enjoying the process and using it as a way to express myself.

At first, I started with other people's recipes. Eventually, I mustered the confidence to create recipes on my own. Now I enjoy mixing and matching flavors and learning what type of ingredients go well together.

Cooking should be about creating. As you allow yourself to experiment in the kitchen, you will feel much more connected to your food and so proud of the winning dishes. Find your inner chef.

Sweet Potato Chips

MAKES 1–2 SERVINGS

♥ **Affirmation:** I am healthy.

Whether we are traveling on the go or need a midday pick-me-up, healthy snacks can give the body the boost of nutrients it needs to keep going. Sweet potatoes are high in vitamin C, vitamin A, calcium, potassium, and beta-carotene, which make them a nutrient-dense food ideal for protecting against the cold and flu as the seasons start to change. Enjoy these chips fresh from the oven, or pack up a bunch and take them with you! Either way, you won't be disappointed.

    1–2 sweet potatoes, peeled

    1 tablespoon olive oil

    2 pinches of sea salt

1. Preheat the oven to 425°F.
2. Cut the potatoes in thin, chiplike slices and remove any extra moisture by patting them with paper towels.
3. Place the oil in a bowl, dip in your fingers, and rub a very light coating of oil over the slices. Place on a baking sheet and sprinkle with the salt.
4. Bake for 10 minutes, then flip the chips. Bake for another 5 to 10 minutes, or until golden brown. Let the chips cool before serving.

Veggie Bites

MAKES 8–16 SERVINGS

♥ **Affirmation:** I embrace curiosity.

Make these snacks with whatever vegetables you like or have on hand in your refrigerator. It's all good!

Coconut oil

2 cups quinoa flour or brown rice flour

Pinch of sea salt

2 eggs, beaten

1 cup veggies, grated or finely chopped

½ cup parsley, finely chopped

1 cup soy milk or rice milk

1. Preheat the oven to 325°F. Lightly coat a mini-muffin pan with the oil.

2. In a medium bowl, stir together the flour and salt. Make a well in the center of the dry ingredients and add the eggs, veggies, and parsley. Stir gently, gradually adding the soy or rice milk. The batter is supposed to be lumpy, so don't overstir.

3. Spoon the batter into the prepared pan. Bake for 12 to 15 minutes. Allow the pan to sit for 10 minutes before removing and serving the bites.

Roasted Cauliflower Mash

MAKES 6–8 SERVINGS

♥ **Affirmation:** I am genuine.

Ever crave the comfort of mashed potatoes? This roasted cauliflower mash will not only trick you into thinking you are eating mashed potatoes but will also provide your body with mood-boosting nutrients and added protein.

1 cauliflower, chopped

1 can (15 ounces) chickpeas, rinsed and drained

½ large onion, chopped

3 garlic cloves

1–2 tablespoons olive oil

Sea salt and ground black pepper

7½ ounces pumpkin puree (from a 15-ounce can)

2 teaspoons pumpkin pie spice

¼ cup almond milk, soy milk, or coconut milk

1 tablespoon maple syrup (optional)

1. Preheat the oven to 350°F.
2. On a large baking sheet, place the cauliflower, chickpeas, onion, and garlic. Lightly coat with the oil. Add salt and pepper to taste. Toss with your hands until all the pieces are coated.
3. Bake for 20 to 25 minutes, or until the cauliflower is golden brown and soft.
4. Transfer the vegetables and excess oil from the baking sheet to a high-powered blender or food processor. Add the pumpkin, pumpkin pie spice, almond or soy or coconut milk, and maple syrup, if using. Process until it forms a smooth mash.
5. Serve immediately, or transfer the mash to a casserole dish and heat for 5 to 10 minutes in the oven before serving.

Cravin' the Crunch Kale Chips

MAKES 1-2 SERVINGS

♥ **Affirmation:** I am abundant.

Sometimes I get the craving for something crunchy. I used to eat entire bags of chips—or leave only four or five chips behind just so I could say I didn't eat the whole bag.

Food shouldn't be a prison. It shouldn't make you feel trapped or bad for eating something.

If I crave something crunchy, kale chips hit just the spot. They crunch, and you can flavor them any way you want. Kale is one of the most nutrient-dense greens and extremely versatile to use. You can bake it, steam it, sauté it, or eat it raw. It helps boost your mood, detoxify your body, and keep you energized all in one serving.

3 bunches kale, stems removed

1-2 tablespoons olive oil

2 pinches of sea salt

Sprinkling of nutritional yeast (optional, for a cheesier flavor)

1. Preheat the oven to 275°F.

2. Spread the kale on a baking sheet. Place the oil in a bowl, dip in your fingers, and rub a very light coating over the kale. Sprinkle on the salt and nutritional yeast, if using.

3. Bake for 25 to 30 minutes, turning the kale halfway through the cooking time, until it turns a bit brown. Watch carefully because it can burn quickly.

Binge-Free Bread Sticks

MAKES 9–12 SERVINGS

♥ **Affirmation:** I accept myself.

Have you ever had a food hangover? Let me define it for you.

Lindsey-ism:

Food hangover (n): When you binge on so much food that the entire night and next morning you feel like you got run over by a truck.

Food hangovers used to happen to me all the time, especially when I'd eat out. My family or friends would order pizza, bread sticks, fried mozzarella cheese sticks, soda, and dessert. I would binge on all the food in front of me because it was "too good" not to eat. The next day, my body paid the toll.

The next time you go out to eat or order out, check in with your body. Are you rushing? Do you notice yourself bingeing? Are you full but you keep eating? Check in with yourself. When you find yourself eating for no reason, start a conversation that gets you excited, have the rest of your meal wrapped to go, and repeat to yourself, "I accept myself."

When you realize you lack nothing, you can always be full.

Olive oil or coconut oil

1 small cauliflower or ½ large cauliflower

2 organic eggs

½ cup mozzarella cheese or vegan cheese

4 tablespoons Italian seasoning

Pinch of sea salt

Pinch of ground black pepper

1. Preheat the oven to 350°F. Lightly coat a baking sheet with the oil.

2. Grate the cauliflower. (I used my food processor and it took about 3 seconds!)

3. In a large bowl, combine the cauliflower, eggs, cheese, Italian seasoning, salt, and pepper. Mix thoroughly.

4. Spread the mixture evenly on the prepared baking sheet. Bake for about 40 minutes, or until golden brown. Cool on a wire rack for 10 to 15 minutes, then cut into strips.

Brussels Sprouts Chips

MAKES 1–2 SERVINGS

♥ **Affirmation:** I embrace new foods.

Growing up, I despised Brussels sprouts. My mom would steam them in the microwave, and I hated the taste.

Recently, I decided to give these guys another try when my mother-in-law served up *roasted* Brussels sprouts at a holiday gathering. They blew my mind! I couldn't believe how much I enjoyed these delicious bites!

Sometimes you experience food in a way that doesn't speak to you or your taste buds. But if you prepare it in another manner or add seasonings, it might become your new favorite food. Be open to food and the possibilities. Try food in various forms, even if you "think" you don't like it. You just might be surprised.

1 cup Brussels sprouts

1 tablespoon olive oil

Sea salt and ground black pepper

1. Preheat the oven to 350°F.

2. Peel the sprouts into layers and place the leaves on a baking sheet. Lightly coat the pieces with the oil. Bake for 7 to 11 minutes, or until crispy. Season with salt and pepper to taste.

Slow It Down Applesauce

MAKES 6–8 SERVINGS

♥ **Affirmation:** I am open to wonder.

Slowing down and taking time to experience the world can open us up to the infinite miracles and wonders the world offers. The same approach applies to eating. When you slow food down and take the time to cook, savor, and experience food and all its flavors, you allow yourself to truly appreciate your food in a deep sense.

This applesauce recipe takes several hours to prepare, which makes it all the more appropriate to slow down and appreciate everything about it. You can savor the aroma as it's cooking, the effort to prepare it, and the ingredients that went into it. Slow things down and enjoy the moment.

12–15 apples (I use a basket of mixed apples)

1 cup water

2 tablespoons fresh lemon juice (1 small lemon)

3 teaspoons ground cinnamon

Ground cloves, ground nutmeg, and cinnamon stick (optional)

1. Peel, core, and cube the apples.

2. Place in a slow cooker with the water and lemon juice. Add the ground cinnamon and the cloves, nutmeg, and cinnamon stick, if desired. Stir everything around. Cover.

3. Cook on low for 4 to 6 hours, checking the consistency every half hour after the fourth hour. To thicken the applesauce, cook with the lid off for the last half hour.

4. Remove the cinnamon stick, if used. With a whisk or an immersion blender, mix the applesauce well. Serve warm or cold.

Date Night Bites

MAKES 1 SERVING

♥ **Affirmation:** I am sweet.

These bites provide the perfect combination of sweet and salty. They also leave your body perfectly balanced, as the sugar from the dates balances with the salt and protein from the nut and cheese. This is a winning combo for any date night or after-dinner treat.

    2 dates

    Small slice of goat cheese

    4 walnut halves

Cut each date in half and remove the pit. Stuff each half with some goat cheese and top with a walnut half. Enjoy!

Lemon Balls

MAKES 12 SERVINGS

♥ **Affirmation:** I am gracious.

Lemon Balls are refreshing and perfect for a midday snack or an after-dinner treat.

    1 cup dates, pitted

    1 cup cashews

    3 tablespoons fresh lemon juice (1 lemon)

    Pinch of sea salt

1. In a blender or food processor, chop the dates. Add the cashews, lemon juice, and salt. Process until the mixture forms one giant ball.
2. Roll the dough into 12 balls. Refrigerate for 1 hour before serving.

Healthy Hot Chocolate

MAKES 1 SERVING

♥ **Affirmation:** I am bubbly.

As winter weather kicks in, our bodies naturally crave warmer foods and drinks such as hot soups and warming teas and ciders. While I am a fan of tea and cider, I also love hot cocoa in the holiday mix. However, most store-bought hot chocolate is filled with chemicals, additives, and tons of sugar. So give your body a break and make your own hot chocolate to ensure its ingredients are few and pure and the taste superb.

   1 cup unsweetened almond milk (or other milk preference)

   1 tablespoon raw cacao powder

   1–2 tablespoons raw or local honey or maple syrup

   1 teaspoon pure vanilla extract

1. In a small saucepan, combine the almond milk and cacao and bring to a small boil. Reduce the heat and whisk until the milk turns a chocolate color. Keep whisking and add in the honey or maple syrup and vanilla.

2. Immediately remove from the heat, pour into a mug, and enjoy!

10

Delectable Desserts

essert is the final sweetness, those moments of pure bliss. When I think of dessert, I think of pleasure.

However, it wasn't always that way. As I discussed in the Introduction, there was a time when I would experience guilt about dessert days *before* attending a picnic or party.

But food (yes, that includes dessert) should be pleasurable. *Food IS pleasurable, but what do you define as pleasure?* Is pleasure bingeing on five pieces of chocolate cake? Or is pleasure enjoying the rich taste, creamy texture, and bountiful flavors of the cake? If you experience healthy pleasure in food, you will digest better, have a better outlook on what you are eating, and feel a sense of satisfaction from one piece rather than five.

I want you to enjoy these desserts with passion, pleasure, and love. Oh, and I want you to feel really good about it. Like really damn good!

Connection Cookies

MAKES 12 COOKIES

♥ **Affirmation:** I feel connected and loved by others.

Sometimes we connect over a cookie. Sometimes we connect over kale. And sometimes it's satisfying enough to just connect and let the experience fill us up. Whichever way, we are craving and seeking connection.

1 cup almond butter

3/4 cup raw or local honey

1 egg

1/4 teaspoon baking soda

Pinch of sea salt

2 cups almond meal

1. Preheat the oven to 350°F.

2. In a large bowl, combine the almond butter, honey, egg, baking soda, and salt. Mix until the egg dissolves and the mixture is smooth and creamy. Slowly add the almond meal until the mixture forms one large ball.

3. Scoop out 12 tablespoon-size balls of dough and place them on a baking sheet. Bake for 10 to 12 minutes, or until the bottoms of the cookies are lightly browned. Let cool before serving with love!

It's Connection That Feeds Us

For years, I carried around much shame and guilt around my food choices, especially as it related to others. Food was one area of my life where I always felt disconnected. I couldn't just go to a party without thinking about food. Would I eat too much? Would I eat too little? Would I be judged for my food choices? If I went to a party, would I automatically binge on cookies?

I constantly rotated through stressful thoughts, such as:

I hope no one sees me eat these cookies. If they do, they probably won't like me.

Ugh, I ate those cookies and now I feel guilty. No one else probably feels like this.

If they see me eat this cookie, they probably won't take me seriously anymore.

In case you can't tell, cookies were my weakness. They were also the one food that tore me apart. They made me feel fat, less than adequate, and disconnected from friends. They were my final frontier: the last remaining food over which I had no self-control.

I felt like the cookies were robbing me of joy. Eventually, however, I realized that it wasn't the cookie at all. This guilt and shame I felt around cookies reflected really a deeper fear of not connecting with people. My stressful thoughts were never about the cookie itself—they reflected the fear that others would judge me.

When it comes down to it, we all want to feel connection: connection with one another, connection with our community, connection with a group, and connection to ourselves.

Connection is what bonds us and gives us a sense of purpose. Connection makes us feel alive. Connection encourages us and shows us that we are not alone.

Connection itself feeds us. It brings us together. It makes us feel full.

Once I recognized that the cookie wasn't to blame, then I needed to embrace a new way of thinking about food. I started seeing those cookies as a symbol of connection and as something that binds us together, not what breaks us apart.

When I made the decision to eat with love and view cookies as a binding force, it drastically changed my relationship with food and my health. I was no longer guilt-tripping about my choices. I was no longer stressing about bingeing. And I no longer felt disconnected from friends and family. I was able to go to a party and feel full from my friendships without the cookie judgments lingering in the back of my mind. And I soon realized that if I wanted to eat a cookie, it was okay. No guilt. No judgments. I just needed to enjoy it and feel good about the community that surrounded me.

So the next time I went to a get-together, I switched from bringing my standard carrot and celery sticks and brought cookies instead. Once I recognized that cookies were not the culprit, I could enjoy one with love and complete connection to others.

PB & Banana Cookies

MAKES 12 COOKIES

♥ **Affirmation:** I am charming.

A great way to cut your processed sugar intake from recipes is to substitute fruits such as unsweetened applesauce, mashed bananas, coconut, dates, and apricots. You can substitute most of these cup for cup. It may take some experimenting! These PB & Banana Cookies hit the spot for a sweet treat without the crash.

Coconut oil

3 ripe bananas, peeled

¼ cup peanut butter

¼ teaspoon baking soda

2 cups oat flour, almond flour, or coconut flour

1. Preheat the oven to 350°F. Lightly coat a baking sheet with the oil.

2. In a blender or food processor, pulse the bananas until they form a paste. Add the peanut butter and baking soda and process until completely smooth. Slowly add in the flour. Process until the dough is moist but not sticky.

3. Roll out 12 teaspoon-size balls and place on the prepared baking sheet. Bake for 10 to 15 minutes, or until golden brown.

Gluten-Free Apple Crisp

MAKES 12 SERVINGS

♥ **Affirmation:** I am caring.

Gluten can be a culprit of mood disorders, so I am always seeking fun and tasty ways to make gluten-free goodies that don't taste like cardboard or Styrofoam. This apple crisp is a simple recipe that doesn't compromise flavor. You can serve it up at a party or make a small batch for a dessert or midday snack.

My husband, Derek, and I had some friends over one week for dinner and dessert. I was in a pinch to make a gluten-free dessert on the fly, so I literally whipped this up 5 minutes before our friends arrived. I had it in and out of the oven and ready to serve by the time dinner was over! This is an awesome holiday dessert that you can feel good about eating.

3 large Granny Smith apples (other apples work, too)

Ground cinnamon

1 cup coconut oil, melted

1/3 cup coconut sugar or raw or local honey (or any natural sweetener you have)

1 1/2 cups almond meal

1. Preheat the oven to 325°F.

2. Cut the apples into cubes and place in an 8 x 10-inch casserole dish. Dust the apples with cinnamon.

3. In a small bowl, combine the oil, sugar or honey, and a few more dashes of cinnamon. Slowly add the almond meal and stir until it is completely mixed in.

4. Spread the mixture evenly over the top of the apples. Sprinkle with a little more cinnamon and drizzle with a little sugar or honey if you wish.

5. Bake for 35 to 40 minutes, or until light brown.

Vegan "Punk"-In Cookies

MAKES 12 COOKIES

♥ **Affirmation:** I love the punk in me!

My husband is a punk rocker. Okay—I know what you are thinking: *What in the heck is Lindsey doing with a punk kid?* Yes, I know. I get that question a lot. In fact, when most people meet him, they are shocked to find out we are married. (Oh, and the same totally goes when his punk friends meet me.)

But to me, punk is about being yourself. It's about honoring your gifts and truly being comfortable in your own skin. And Derek is the perfect example of someone who stands firmly in who he is. I admire that about him. So I made him these cookies to celebrate him being himself. And just know—there's a bit of punk in all of us!

Coconut oil

½ cup pumpkin puree

½ cup almond butter

¼ cup coconut sugar or agave nectar

1 tablespoon pumpkin pie spice

1½ cups almond meal

¼ cup vegan chocolate chips

1. Preheat the oven to 425°F. Lightly coat a baking sheet with the oil.

2. In a large bowl, combine the puree, almond butter, sugar or nectar, and pumpkin pie spice. Stir until creamy. Slowly add the almond meal and stir until the batter forms a large ball and is easy to shape. (Depending on the moisture content of the other ingredients, you may need to add extra almond meal to get the right consistency.) Stir in the chips.

3. Roll pieces of the dough into 12 tablespoon-size balls and press them down on the prepared baking sheet. Bake for 10 to 12 minutes, or until the bottoms are lightly browned. Let cool before serving.

No-Bake Chocolate Pie

MAKES 8 SERVINGS

♥ **Affirmation:** I am not alone. I am connected to community.

The shame behind our eating is usually a deeper fear of not being able to connect with others. We think, *No one struggles this hard with food like I do.* Or *I am the only one thinking about that chocolate pie right now.* Or *Why can't I get my eating under control?*

At the end of the day, we all want to feel connected. If we're busy feeling that we are the only person struggling with food or dealing with emotional eating issues, we can't connect to the group as a whole. Just remember that you are not alone. We all have unique relationships with food, and there are so many others experiencing similar feelings.

Create this chocolate pie with the intention that we are all connected. Savor each bite for its rich flavor. And feel the connection of people around you.

1 cup cashews

15–20 pitted dates

1/2 cup coconut oil, melted

3/4 cup coconut nectar, raw or local honey, or another natural liquid sweetener

1 tablespoon pure vanilla extract

Pinch of sea salt

2 cups raw cacao powder

1. In a blender or food processor, pulse the cashews and dates until the mixture forms a solid ball of dough. Pat the dough evenly into an ungreased pie pan. Set this crust aside.

2. In a medium bowl, combine the oil, sweetener, vanilla, and salt. Stir a few times. Slowly add the cacao and mix until the powder is completely dissolved.

3. Slowly pour the chocolate into the pie crust and spread evenly. Refrigerate up to 20 minutes before serving.

Confidence Clusters

MAKES 12 CLUSTERS

♥ **Affirmation:** I am confident.

Nuts are a great mood-boosting food that also improve blood circulation, which in turn can help clear your mind and give you a boost in confidence. If you are headed out for a night on the town and want to give your body a mental boost, make a batch of Confidence Clusters! They are sweet enough to curb a sugar craving and filling enough to keep you satisfied.

1 cup almonds, chopped

1 cup pecans, chopped

⅓ cup raw or local honey

⅓ cup peanut butter

1. In a medium bowl, stir the almonds and pecans. Set aside.

2. In a small bowl, combine the honey and peanut butter. Slowly add the honey mixture to the nuts. Scrape the mixture into a small casserole dish and refrigerate for 1 hour.

3. When set, cut into 12 small bars or random shapes for clusters.

Chunky Monkey Ice Cream

MAKES 1 SERVING

♥ **Affirmation:** I choose to laugh and smile today!

There's no cream in this ice cream—just a deliciously creamy texture that will put a grin on your face! Make the recipe easier by cutting the banana into chunks before freezing it.

1 banana, peeled and frozen

½ cup almond milk, coconut milk, or rice milk

1 tablespoon peanut butter

1 tablespoon dark chocolate chips or dairy-free chocolate chips

1. In a blender or food processor, combine the banana, almond or coconut or rice milk, and peanut butter until smooth and creamy.

2. Place the mixture in a bowl, top with the chocolate chips, and dig in!

making mischief

Eating ice cream reminds me of being a little kid. I think it's important for all of us to embrace our childlike tendencies and to act playful, be mischievous, and laugh.

Of course, you don't always need to eat ice cream to feel like a kid again. Here are nonfood ways to re-create childlike tendencies:

- Watch your favorite childhood movie. Do you remember how you felt watching it? Capture those feelings again!

- Drink out of a silly straw.

- Play your favorite childhood board game with friends and family.

- Laugh and smile. Don't take life so seriously!

Chocolate Chip Quinoa Cookies

MAKES 12 COOKIES

♥ **Affirmation:** My body is strong and powerful.

These quick and easy quinoa cookies are high in protein and easy to digest. They can make either a healthy sweet treat or an easy on-the-go breakfast. (Yes, you heard right—this dessert can also be consumed as a breakfast!)

1 cup quinoa, rinsed well

3/4 cup quick-cooking or rolled oats

1/2 teaspoon sea salt

1 tablespoon ground cinnamon

2 tablespoons maple syrup

1/2 cup almond butter

1/2 cup dark chocolate chips

1. Preheat the oven to 350°F.

2. Cook the quinoa according to package directions. Let cool. Measure out 2 cups of the cooked quinoa; save any remainder for another recipe or meal.

3. In a large bowl, combine the oats, salt, and cinnamon. Add the cooled quinoa, maple syrup, almond butter, and chocolate chips. Mix well.

4. Scoop into 1-inch round balls and place on a nonstick baking sheet. Bake for 20 minutes, or until the bottoms are lightly browned. Let cool and enjoy!

Crunchy Bliss Bites

MAKES 12 BALLS

♥ **Affirmation:** I am blissful.

Do you make a run for the fridge at 8:00 at night? Do you have an "emergency" chocolate bar hidden in your desk drawer? When you find yourself reaching for food during these times, ask yourself: What you are really hungry for? Oftentimes, we seek comfort in food when really we need nourishment from other areas of our lives. So when you find yourself headed to the fridge, try to determine what you really need emotionally.

½ cup cashews

¼ cup coconut shreds

¾ cup quick-cooking oats

1 teaspoon sea salt

2 tablespoons raw cacao powder

6 teaspoons coconut oil

2 teaspoons raw or local honey

½ cup almond butter

1. In a blender or food processor, pulse the cashews and coconut until fine. (For a little crunch in the finished cookie, process a little less.)

2. Transfer to a bowl and add the oats, salt and cacao. Stir. Add the oil and mix. Gradually mix in the honey and almond butter until the mixture forms a ball.

3. Take pieces of the dough and roll into 12 little balls. Chill for 2 hours before serving. Store in an airtight container for up to 1 week.

TIP: Freeze the bites for a late-night sweet craving without the guilt!

Chia Seed Pudding

MAKES 4 SERVINGS

♥ **Affirmation:** I am relaxed.

Chi, chi, chi, chia! Yes, these little chia seeds are the same seeds used on those Chia Pets you'd see on TV infomercials. However, don't let the little pets fool you. Chia seeds, in natural form, are quite the plant-based powerhouse. Just 1 tablespoon of chia seeds provides 6 grams of fiber, 3 grams of protein, and 3 grams of omega-3 fatty acids.

You can add chia seeds to smoothies or even use them as sprinkles on cold treats. Even better, try this delicious chocolate chia seed pudding. It's a crossbreed between a tapioca pudding and chocolate pudding, without all the added fillers.

1 cup unsweetened almond milk or coconut milk

2 tablespoons raw cacao powder

¼ cup chia seeds

¼ cup maple syrup

1. In a small bowl, combine the almond or coconut milk and cacao, stirring until the cacao is blended in. Add the chia seeds and maple syrup and mix well.

2. Place the bowl in the refrigerator and chill for 2 to 3 hours, or until set.

Chocovado Mousse

♥ **Affirmation:** I am beautiful, inside and out.

While preparing this recipe for a delicious chocolate and avocado mousse, I stopped to recognize the beauty of its fruits. An avocado has a thick outside layer, but when you open it, the center is soft and creamy. The soft green color makes the avocado special and unique. The banana also has a firm outside layer and a creamy middle. It's sweet and tasty and can be used for a multitude of purposes.

Aren't these fruits kind of like people? We have hard, exterior shells to protect us from disease and infection, yet inside we are soft and unique. It's important to recognize your own beauty every time you get a chance. When you make this mousse, take a minute to appreciate and love your unique attributes.

1 avocado

1 banana (preferably frozen)

½ cup almond milk or rice milk

1 tablespoon raw cacao powder

½ tablespoon raw or local honey

Ice cubes (optional)

In a blender, combine the avocado, banana, almond or rice milk, cacao, and honey until smooth. Add ice for a thicker texture, if desired. Serve immediately.

Almond Butter Tartlets

MAKES 12 TARTLETS

♥ **Affirmation:** I release judgment and perfectionism from my life.

These layered tartlets remind me of the layers we all have. Sometimes it takes some hard work, digesting and understanding our inner selves, to uncover these deeper issues around food. Once we uncover and address them, we can truly feel freedom from food and experience the richness life has to offer.

Almond Filling

1½ cups raw almonds

2 tablespoons maple syrup

Smooth Chocolate

⅓ cup coconut oil, room temperature or melted

¼ cup maple syrup

1 teaspoon pure vanilla extract

1 cup raw cacao powder

1. Line one 12-cup muffin pan with paper liners.
2. To make the almond filling: In a blender or food processor, combine the almonds and maple syrup until smooth but still gritty. Set aside.
3. To make the smooth chocolate: In a large bowl, combine the oil, maple syrup, and vanilla. Slowly add in the cacao and mix until smooth and creamy.
4. Take out half of the smooth chocolate and place it in a medium bowl. Slowly add in about ¼ cup almond filling. Scoop 12 tablespoon-size balls of this chocolate-almond mixture into the paper liners. Press until the bottom of the liner is covered with chocolate.
5. Next, place 1 tablespoon of the almond filling in each muffin cup and spread evenly.
6. Finally, top off the tarts with a layer of the remaining smooth chocolate.
7. Refrigerate for up to 1 hour, or until the chocolate hardens. Keep refrigerated.

what Is Your Food saying about Your Life?

How you view food probably reflects a lot about how you view life.

Think about it: Are you someone who eats and eats yet never feels satisfied? Or someone who is always hungry? If you feel a lack about food, you probably feel a lack about life.

You are probably someone who also never feels good enough. Maybe you never feel you are doing enough. Or will never be successful enough. The lack in food is a reflection of the lack you feel in life.

Think about your deeper food story. Is it shaping who you are today? If so, what perfectionisms or fears are holding you back? How can you gain the support and confidence to move forward?

Cookie Dough Bites

MAKES 12 BALLS

♥ Affirmation: I am fun!

As a kid, I was obsessed with licking cookie dough batter from the mixing bowl. However, my mom warned me that I could get salmonella poisoning from the raw eggs, so it always made me a bit anxious to sneak batter. But come on, it's really the best part of the cookie-making process! So I came up with egg-free Cookie Dough Bites that taste just like the batter. You can freeze them for a cool summer treat or serve them as is to friends and family.

½ cup almond butter

⅓ cup raw or local honey or maple syrup

1 cup almond flour or cashew flour

¼ cup chocolate chips

1. Combine the almond butter and honey or maple syrup. Add the nut flour and mix until a ball of dough forms. Add the chocolate chips.

2. Roll into 12 bite-size balls and freeze for 30 minutes.

Fearless Cookies

MAKES 12 COOKIES

♥ **Affirmation:** I am fearless and free.

Fear is the thing that holds us back, that paralyzes our minds and keeps us from taking the next step. I used to fear baking. In fact, I always said that I could never bake. The truth is, the only baking I did came from a box cookie mix to which you add water. Even so, I always managed to burn the cookies!

I decided to face my fear of baking with simple recipes. Once I got the formulas and methods down, my confidence grew. Before long, I could whip up baked goods that were healthy and delicious.

Sometimes it takes facing our fears to recognize that we have the power, the strength, and the intelligence to overcome any obstacle put in our path. The moment we overcome fear is the moment our freedom journey begins.

1 cup almond butter

¾ cup raw or local honey

1 egg

¼ teaspoon baking soda

Pinch of sea salt

2 cups almond meal

1. Preheat the oven to 350°F.

2. In a large bowl, combine the almond butter, honey, egg, baking soda, and salt. Mix until the egg is completely incorporated and the mixture is smooth and creamy. Slowly add the almond meal until a solid dough ball forms.

3. Scoop out 12 tablespoon-size balls of dough and place them on a baking sheet. Bake for 10 to 12 minutes, or until the bottoms of the cookies are lightly browned. Let cool and serve with love!

11

Body Love

t's so important to not only nourish yourself physically but also emotionally. The tools, tips, and recipes in this chapter move beyond food. They nourish our skin, our bodies, our minds, and our souls.

Many of my own experiences with food were really the tragic results of not feeling good enough about myself, full enough emotionally, or satisfied mentally. I thought a flatter tummy would fix my issues, but I soon realized that body love has to be enjoyed at all stages in life.

So I Got Called Fat

I was having a deep conversation with a friend and I opened up about some insecurities that I used to have about my body. I mentioned how I've never been superskinny and that when I first started health coaching, I was worried people weren't going to take me seriously since the whole "skinny = healthy" thing is stuck in our minds. As our conversation unfolded, my friend mentioned that someone had indeed once told her I must be a bad food coach because I wasn't skinny enough.

At first, I wasn't surprised by this response; after all, I'd been telling myself that for years. But to hear it from someone else for the first time—well, it's a tough pill to swallow.

Then my mind started racing. I thought, *Wait, am I a bad coach? No, they are just insecure. Should I get really skinny and prove to the world that I can do it?*

Part of me laughed about it and the other part of me was almost in tears.

The fact is—I am not skinny. The truth is—I once struggled with an eating disorder. Usually after I emotionally binged on something to mask my insecurities about my weight and body, I would self-induce a panic attack so I could throw up in the bathroom.

I was paralyzed by the road society paved: that women have to be skinny in order to be beautiful and wanted. (Let's face it—it only takes skimming one issue of *Maxim* magazine to make you feel bad about yourself.) Because of this, my inner mean girl kept saying the same thing over and over again: "If you aren't skinny, you are worthless."

For many others, the voice can also show up and say things like:

- If you don't have a six-pack, you aren't trying hard enough.

- If you are too skinny, you are anorexic and sick.

- If you are too white, you are pasty.

The list seriously goes on and on and on.

In all of this, we spend so much time checking in with the outside world, we forget to check in with ourselves. We care so much about others' thoughts and insecurities that we put our own aside. We let others define us. And the moment we let others define us is the moment we lose ourselves.

I will admit it, I lost myself for a while. Dieting days on end. Obsessively worrying about the number on a scale. Insecure in my being. Ashamed of going in public. Suffering from social anxiety. Uncomfortable in all of my clothes. And constantly comparing myself to everyone around me. *(Wait, are they skinnier than me?)*

My body became a puppet that someone else was directing, telling me how to move, what to say, and how to act.

Let's start cutting the strings and performing our own show for once. Here are some "recipes" to cut the ties and be more of who you are.

Throw Out the Scale

♥ **Affirmation:** I define me!

1. Take the scale out of your bathroom (or other area of your house).

2. Throw it in the trash, donate it, or recycle it.

3. Don't buy a new scale.

Seriously. Throw it out. Smash it. Donate it. Get rid of it. A scale does not define you. Stop relying on a number to tell you that you are worthy, beautiful, fit enough, good enough, brave enough, or perfect enough. You are enough, just the way you are.

Quit Comparing

♥ **Affirmation:** I embrace being me.

1. Notice when you compare yourself to others.

2. STOP IT!

Quit comparing yourself to friends, family, celebrities, and strangers. Actress Jamie Lee Curtis has an expression that I love: "Compare and despair!" Comparison kills, literally. Get off Facebook for a day if you find yourself scrolling and comparing. Get outside. Connect with nature. Embrace the qualities that you love about yourself. Be around people who uplift you. Do more of what you love.

Recognize the BS

♥ **Affirmation:** I lift up myself and others.

1. Recognize your negative thoughts.

2. Recognize that everyone else has these same negative thoughts.

3. STOP and realize we are in this together.

4. Repeat.

Recognize the BS! Seriously, everyone deals with this crap. I am no different. We all think these thoughts. We all have those moments. I don't care if you are Gandhi, Mother Teresa, or the next big guru in health and wellness—these insecurities creep in from time to time. We are in this together. And we need to collectively start changing our views when it comes to health and beauty. We need to pave a new road of norms and quit following the broken, shallow, and empty path we've been continuously led down. Practice lifting other women up. Check your words. Say nice things. Be kind.

Embrace You!

♥ **Affirmation:** I embrace me!

1. List good things about yourself.

2. Repeat often.

Find the qualities that are good in *you*! Take a minute to write five things that you absolutely love about yourself. Don't be shy—brag a little!

1. _____

2. _____

3. _____

4. _____

5. _____

Practice Simple Meditation

♥ **Affirmation:** I love my body the way it is.

1. Sit down.

2. Breathe.

3. Repeat an affirmation.

You don't have to sit on a rock and close your eyes for hours to experience meditation. Make meditation simple: Sit in an upright position and with your feet planted on the floor. Close your eyes. Breathe in through your nose and exhale from your mouth. Continue breathing until it becomes easy. Then repeat the affirmation, "I love my body the way it is." Repeat ten times. Continue focusing on your breath. Place your hand on your heart and thank your body. Open your eyes and come back to the space. Appreciate yourself for taking the time to complete a simple meditation.

Practice Makeup-Free Monday (or Any Day of the Week)

♥ **Affirmation:** I love the skin I'm in.

1. Wake up.

2. Don't put makeup on.

3. Do something you love.

4. Feel happy.

The moment I realized that I was literally painting my face full of chemicals each day is the moment I lost it. I later found out that women spend about 137 days of their life getting ready. And for what? Sure, dressing up every now and then can make us feel empowered and good. But to go to the grocery store with a full painted face is a bit much.

So I thought, what if we went makeup-free one day a week and focused that hour on doing something that we loved and cared about? We are always finding excuses not to do something that makes us happy, so why not ditch our makeup time and do something we love? This will feed your soul and give your skin a break!

Body Nourishments to Make

Can you be makeup-free and still pamper your body? Absolutely. Loving your body is about choosing to nourish it in a way that expresses the highest quality and love. What you put on your skin is just as important as what you put in your body!

Here are some simple products you can prepare at home to give your skin the very best TLC.

Love Your Skin Scrub

MAKES 1 APPLICATION

♥ **Affirmation:** I am already sweet enough.

Your skin is your largest organ—it needs some body love from time to time, too! Using body products made without toxic chemicals can make you feel more in tune with nature and more connected to what's not only going *in* your body but what's going *on* top of it!

1 tablespoon raw sugarcane crystals

3 tablespoons raw or local honey

1½ tablespoons fresh lemon juice (½ lemon)

1. Combine the sugar, honey, and lemon juice, mixing well with a spoon. Make sure the consistency is thick, not runny.

2. Wash your hands, then apply the mixture on your clean face. Scrub for 30 to 45 seconds, then remove with warm water.

Pearly White Glow

MAKES 1 APPLICATION

♥ **Affirmation:** I am smiling and happy.

Use this tooth treatment only one or two times a month. This is not meant to be an everyday toothpaste!

2 tablespoons baking soda

2 tablespoons hydrogen peroxide

1 tablespoon sea salt

3-ounce glass or plastic container

1. Combine the baking soda, hydrogen peroxide, and salt in the small container.
2. Place the mixture on your toothbrush and gently go over your teeth. Avoid getting it on your gums—especially if you have sensitive teeth. Let it sit for a minute, then rinse.

To the Tip of Your Tongue

After you eat, pieces of leftover food remain on your tongue. This can make your taste buds more susceptible to craving the type of food you recently ate. Using a tongue cleaner (also known as a tongue scraper or tongue brush) is a great way to clear your taste buds so you are less susceptible to cravings. It also helps freshen the breath and makes food taste better. Both your dentist and your significant other will thank you!

Cleansing Shampoo

MAKES 2–4 APPLICATIONS

♥ **Affirmation:** Cleaning heals me.

Is there anything more uplifting than shiny clean locks?! An empty travel bottle makes an ideal container for this shampoo.

    ½ cup water

    3 tablespoons baking soda

    4–6 drops tea tree oil

    Small glass or plastic bottle

1. Place the water, baking soda, and oil in the bottle and shake well.
2. Squirt some shampoo onto your hair, lather, and let it sit about a minute. Then rinse thoroughly.

Craving-Kicker Mist

MAKES 120 SPRAYS

♥ **Affirmation:** I am divine.

Spritz and breathe in this spray whenever you feel a craving come on.

    3-ounce glass or plastic spray bottle

    Distilled water

    5–7 drops ylang-ylang essential oil

    5–7 drops orange essential oil

    5–7 drops bergamot essential oil

    5–7 drops lemon essential oil

Fill the bottle three-quarters of the way up with the distilled water. Add the essential oils. Shake before using.

Calming Pillow Spray

MAKES 120 SPRAYS

♥ **Affirmation:** I am grateful for this day.

Apply five sprays of this soothing spray on your pillow before you go to bed. With each spritz, think of something you have to be grateful for that day.

   3-ounce glass or plastic spray bottle

   Distilled water

   30 drops lavender essential oil

   20 drops lemon essential oil

Fill the bottle three-quarters of the way up with the distilled water. Add the essential oils. Shake before using.

In Conclusion: Your Body Is Amazing

Congratulations for reaching this point, and thank you for journeying with me through stories, recipes, and lots of inspiration in between. Everyone has a unique journey, including you! Where you are now is not where you will be in two days, two years, or twenty years.

But there's one thing I hope you remember as you go forward. And this is it: *your body is fricking amazing.*

It breathes without reminders to do so.

It beats a heartbeat to keep you alive.

It heals even the deepest wounds.

It grows your hair back from a bad haircut.

It energizes you to run, play, and laugh.

It feels deeply and intimately.

It protects you from outside harm.

It digests food to keep you sustained all day long.

It even digests junk food. (Yup, even that slice of triple-chocolate cake.)

So let's face it—*your body is a magical machine that is constantly working for you and through you.*

While you've been shaming your body in the bathroom mirror or smack-talking your thighs to a friend, your body has been doing everything in its power to save you, nourish you, protect you, and keep you alive.

It literally fights for your life, every single day.

The next time you catch yourself about to bad-mouth your body, stop, take a deep breath, and express gratitude for all the things your body is doing daily to keep your heart beating.

And then you can realize why there is absolutely nothing wrong with you or your body.

Relinquish your food guilt, love your body, and eat your way to happiness.

Index